Accession no.
36097414

ON BEREAVEMENT

D0293211

FACING DEATH

Series editor: David Clark, Professor of Medical Sociology,
University of Sheffield

The subject of death in late modern culture has become a rich field of theoretical, clinical and policy interest. Widely regarded as a taboo until recent times, death now engages a growing interest among social scientists, practitioners and those responsible for the organization and delivery of human services. Indeed, how we die has become a powerful commentary on how we live and the specialized care of dying people holds an important place within modern health and social care.

This series captures such developments. Among the contributors are leading experts in death studies, from sociology, anthropology, social psychology, ethics, nursing, medicine and pastoral care. A particular feature of the series is its attention to the developing field of palliative care, viewed from the perspectives of practitioners, planners and policy analysts; here several authors adopt a multidisciplinary approach, drawing on recent research, policy and organizational commentary, and reviews of evidence-based practice. Written in a clear, accessible style, the entire series will be essential reading for students of death, dying and bereavement and for anyone with an involvement in palliative care research, service delivery or policy making.

Current and forthcoming titles:

David Clark, Jo Hockley, Sam Ahmedzai (eds): *New Themes in Palliative Care*
David Clark and Jane E. Seymour: *Reflections on Palliative Care*
Mark Cobb: *The Dying Soul: Spiritual Care at the End of Life*
Kirsten Costain Schou and Jenny Hewison: *Experiencing Cancer: Quality of Life in Treatment*
Catherine Exley: *Living with Cancer, Living with Dying*
David Field, David Clark, Jessica Corner and Carol Davis (eds): *Researching Palliative Care*
Jenny Hockey, Jeanne Katz and Neil Small (eds): *Grief, Mourning and the Death Ritual*
David Kissane and Sidney Bloch: *Family Grief Therapy*
Gordon Riches and Pamela Dawson: *An Intimate Loneliness: Supporting Bereaved Parents and Siblings*
Jane E. Seymour: *Critical Moments: Death and Dying in Intensive Care*
Tony Walter: *On Bereavement: The Culture of Grief*

ON BEREAVEMENT
The culture of grief

TONY WALTER

LIS - LIBRARY

Date	Fund
04/05/10	n

Order No.

WITHDRAWN
2106097

University of Chester

OPEN UNIVERSITY PRESS
Maidenhead · Philadelphia

Open University Press
McGraw-Hill Education
McGraw-Hill House
Shoppenhangers Road
Maidenhead
Berkshire
England
SL6 2QL

email: enquiries@openup.co.uk
world wide web: www.openup.co.uk

and
Two Penn Plaza,
New York, NY 10121-2289, USA

First Published 1999
Reprinted 2001, 2010

Copyright © Tony Walter, 1999

All rights reserved. Except for the quotation of short passages for the
purpose of criticism and review, no part of this publication may be
reproduced, stored in a retrieval system, or transmitted, in any form or
by any means, electronic, mechanical, photocopying, recording or otherwise,
without the prior written permission of the publisher or a licence from the
Copyright Licensing Agency Limited. Details of such licences (for reprographic
reproduction) may be obtained from the Copyright Licensing Agency Ltd of
90 Tottenham Court Road, London, W1P 0LP.

A catalogue record of this book is available from the British Library

ISBN 978 0 335 20081 8 (hb)   978 0 335 20080 1 (pb)

Library of Congress Cataloging-in-Publication Data
Walter, Tony. 1948–
    On bereavement : the culture of grief / Tony Walter.
        p.   cm. — (Facing death)
    Includes bibliographical references and index.
    ISBN 0–335–20081–8. — ISBN 0–335–20080–X (pbk.)
    1. Death—Social aspects.   2. Bereavement—Social aspects.
3. Thanatology.   I. Title.   II. Series.
HO1073.W36   1999
306.9—dc21   99–13298
                                                                            CIP

Typeset by Graphicraft Limited, Hong Kong
Printed in Great Britain by Bell & Bain Ltd, Glasgow

for
Liz, Hannah and Jack

Contents

Series editor's preface   ix
Acknowledgements   xii
Introduction   xiii

Prologue   1

Part I Living with the dead   17
Introduction to Part I   19

  1 Other places, other times   23
  2 War, peace and the dead: twentieth-century popular culture   39
  3 Private bonds   56
  4 Public bonds: the dead in everyday conversation   69
  5 The last chapter   84
  6 Theories   103

Part II Policing grief   117
Introduction to Part II   119

  7 Guidelines for grief: historical background   127
  8 Popular guidelines: the English case   138
  9 Expert guidelines: clinical lore   154
10 Vive la différence? The politics of gender   168
11 Bereavement care   185

12 Conclusion: integration, regulation and postmodernism   205

References   209
Index   225

Series editor's preface

Tony Walter has produced a most welcome fourth contribution to the Facing Death series. Whilst earlier writers in the series have concentrated upon developments in palliative care (Clark, Hockley and Ahmedzai 1998; Clark and Seymour 1999) and upon the 'treatment calendars' associated with experiencing cancer (Costain Schou and Hewison 1999), now we have a book which moves beyond the dying process and death itself, to focus on the phenomenon of *bereavement*. In so doing Tony Walter has produced the most sustained sociological analysis yet of this complex and multifaceted subject.

Of course, the closing decades of the twentieth century saw innumerable books on bereavement. Indeed, as Walter shows, these formed part of an entire intellectual and clinical paradigm whereby the experiences of loss, grief and mourning were fixed within a predominantly psychological set of understandings and interventions. In this book such writings are treated as a topic rather more than a resource. Walter brings to bear a sociological questioning which is eager to uncover the conditions which made possible the rise and eventual ascendancy of the psychological paradigm, to link this to the preoccupations of late modern culture, and to say something of its consequences for bereaved people, for those who 'work' with them and for the dead themselves.

He is able to do this so successfully by adopting both a historical and a comparative perspective on his subject matter. As readers we are thus happily denied that pervasive double fallacy of the modern world which would have us believe that there is no time but the present and no place but here. Accordingly, the whole of the first part of this book is concerned with the ways in which human societies – traditional, modern, post-modern – engage with and relate to their dead. Through a close examination of the anthropological literature we are able to explore the prospects of societies which may either under- or over-integrate their dead members. This in turn provides a key to one of the central themes of this book, which examines how our social relationship to the dead may tell us something about the very business of living itself. It is in such ways that Walter draws so helpfully on the ideas of the great French sociologist of a century ago, Emile Durkheim.

By giving so much priority to *culture* as a framework within which we can understand bereavement and grief, Walter is able to resist defining his subject solely within the parameters of medical and caring discourses. He gives attention to the importance of war in the twentieth century as a source of multiple bereavement reactions and social responses shaped by nation, generation and gender. He also encourages us to think anew about the social and cultural responses to death which occur in times of comparative peace. In this way the social significances of both 'remembering' and 'forgetting' the dead are enunciated. In modern culture in peacetime, it is 'forgetting', of course, which has tended to predominate, at least in public. Remembering the dead thus becomes a private matter, which in some marginalized forms may attract opprobrium or scorn.

Making sense of all of this calls for theoretical frameworks and a discussion of these forms the bridge into Part II of the book, where Walter turns his attention to various ways in which grief can be seen to be 'policed' in modern societies. Central to this are ideas about the reflexive nature of identity in the modern world, so that fitting together a picture of the dead, as Walter puts it, 'is therefore made necessary yet impeded by modern conditions' (p.82). One of the ways in which we do this is through the construction of some sort of narrative of 'the good death', and it is very useful again to be reminded in Tony Walter's excellent Chapter 5, that this notion extends well beyond its current usage in the palliative care movement.

The account of theories of bereavement which is presented here will make vital reading for students and practitioners in this field. It takes us from Freud to the 'new' bereavement theories and in particular shows how a 'clinical lore' has developed which emphasizes that for bereaved people the breaking of affectional bonds with the dead is the necessary route to 'adjustment'. It is this 'clinical lore', together with its theoretical underpinnings which forms the foundation for modern methods of 'policing grief'. Walter's approach to this issue is challenging and imaginative. He is not out to undermine the authority and endeavours of grief practitioners. Indeed he describes his own 'third way' orientation to the field of bereavement counselling, which he treats as a topic of enquiry but seeks neither to attack nor promote.

Again, this is a discussion which benefits from a historical perspective, as in Chapter 7 where we are shown how the regulation of emotions of grief has been altering since the sixteenth century. The English case serves as a particular illustration of this and no less than seven different 'scripts' or grieving norms are identified: personal, anomic, private, forbidden, time-limited, distracted and expressive. From here Walter returns to his theme of 'clinical lore' and the primacy of 'working through' painful emotions as the leitmotif in clinical practice. Some insight is offered here into the ways in which 'descriptions' produced by researchers may quickly become the 'prescriptions' of practitioners. The tricky concept of 'normal grief' is at the heart of much of this, and this as Walter shows in the following chapter, is a matter of some variation between men and women. There follows a discussion of bereavement care and bereavement services and it is noted how little researched these are by sociologists and those who use qualitative methods.

Tony Walter concludes his book by showing how our understanding of contemporary grief is shaped by the twin axes of *integration* and *regulation*. Modern bereavement is thus a product of the extent to which we let go of the dead, or maintain continuing bonds. It is also governed by whether the feelings associated with grief are actively expressed, or specifically contained. There will be much in this to stimulate the thinking of those who, hitherto, have been unaware of the potential for sociological thinking on this subject.

This book on bereavement will be followed by some related titles in the Facing Death series: other works by Gordon Riches and Pamela Dawson, by Jenny Hockey, Jeanne Katz and Neil Small, and by David Kissane and Sydney Bloch will soon follow. Tony Walter must be congratulated however on producing a sociological book on bereavement which is the product of such wide reading and imaginative analysis. I predict that this book will have a considerable readership and that those already familiar with the initial work of Tony Walter on bereavement will be further inspired and stimulated by this full length exploration.

David Clark

References

Clark, D., Hockey, J. and Ahmedzai, S. (1998) *New Themes in Palliative Care*. Buckingham: Open University Press.

Clark, D. and Seymour, J. (1999) *Reflections on Palliative Care*. Buckingham: Open University Press.

Costain Schou, K. and Hewison, J. (1999) *Experiencing Cancer*. Buckingham: Open University Press.

Acknowledgements

I would like to thank David Clark for inviting me to write this book. My thanks also to David Clark, Dennis Klass, Jan McLaren, Colin Murray Parkes and Margaret Stroebe for their helpful, and in two cases exceptionally detailed, comments on early drafts. I hope I have dealt with your comments with the same care you have given my drafts. I am indebted to Gordon Riches for the idea of developing a Durkheimian approach to bereavement, though whether he would recognize what I have come up with is another matter! I also thank the interviewee who appears in the Prologue.

Chapter 1 includes material from the forthcoming chapter by Dennis Klass and myself in Stroebe *et al.*'s (forthcoming) *New Handbook of Bereavement*. Chapters 4 and 5 discuss and expand the ideas contained in my 1996 article, 'A new model of grief' (Walter 1996b). Chapter 8 updates my 1997 chapter, 'Emotional reserve and the English way of grief' (Walter 1997a).

Introduction

The social world of bereavement is currently undergoing conflict and change. Strangely, very little of the rapidly growing literature on bereavement has examined this. Although the mourner as a social being may be found in studies of other cultures and in historical studies of our own past, most literature on bereavement in the modern West depicts only isolated individuals, at most individuals in families, dealing with their own private grief. Somehow, other people, culture and the dead themselves all get missed out, even though those who are bereaved often find other people, culture and the dead as much of an issue as their own inner psychological journey. This book attempts to redress this imbalance in two ways.

Letting go, keeping hold

First, the dominant idea of the twentieth century has been that grief is eventually 'resolved' by 'detaching', 'letting go' and 'moving on' to new relationships. The last decade of the century, however, has witnessed a sustained assault on this idea, both by academic researchers and by bereaved people themselves (by no means two mutually exclusive groups). Study after study has documented that while some do indeed leave the dead behind, many others maintain a bond with their dead indefinitely, even while forging new social ties. They do not let go and move on; they transform the relationship, keep hold and move on. Others, primarily elderly with little time themselves left on this earth, have no intention of letting go; they hold on to their memories, waiting to join their beloved in the hereafter. I have lost count of the number of times people have expressed relief when they have been told that it is all right to keep hold of the dead person, rather than to leave them behind. Clearly, whatever their inner experience, bereaved people live in a social context that promotes some ideas of grieving and pathologizes others; these ideas in part shape the bereaved person's experience.

Bereavement typically entails both an urge to stay with the dead and an urge to get on with life (Stroebe and Schut 1999). Societies have varied as to which urge they have legitimated. Nineteenth-century romanticism, for example, legitimated the urge to stay with the dead (at least for women), twentieth-century modernism urged us to leave the past and the dead behind and look to the future, while end-of-millennium postmodernism encourages a diversity in which both urges may be allowed (Stroebe *et al.* 1992).

I will not waste space arguing the case for continuing bonds, for it is already well established (see Klass *et al.* 1996). My aim in Part I is rather to flesh out the case by exploring some ways in which the living and the dead interact in contemporary western cultures. Crucially, I show that this interaction is not just within the head of the individual bereaved person, but is part and parcel of how families and indeed entire societies keep in touch with their past, and thus with their present and their future. Bereavement has to do with group history as well as with individual psychology.

Culture

Second, this book breaks new ground by exploring the influence of mainline culture on how people grieve in modern western countries, notably Britain and the United States of America. There are a number of publications (e.g. Irish *et al.* 1993; Parkes *et al.* 1997) that document cultural prescriptions for mourning, but, with very few exceptions (such as Kalish and Reynolds 1981; Eisenbruch 1984), they ignore mainline white culture. It is as though 'other' cultures need explaining, whereas mainline white culture does not (Klass, forthcoming). Indeed, this is precisely how a number of nurses, funeral directors and other workers perceive things; they request fact-files and succinct articles describing the funeral and mourning traditions of Sikhs, Jews, Hindus and other groups that they, from time to time, are called to serve. This burgeoning literature not only gives the misleading impression that each minority culture is unitary and static rather than diverse and changing (Gunaratnam 1997), but also reinforces the impression that the mainline white culture of mourning is unproblematic.

Many other books and articles, however, bemoan the contemporary culture of grief, blaming it for exacerbating the experience of bereavement today – if only we still had the rituals of past times or other cultures, they assert, grief would not be half so bad. Yet despite the promising start made by Gorer (1965), there is hardly any literature that carefully examines the contemporary mainstream white culture of mourning, how it has evolved and how it is currently in ferment. Although we now have the beginnings of a history of twentieth-century wartime bereavement (Winter 1995; Bourke 1996), no one seems to have contemplated writing a history of twentieth-century peacetime bereavement.

Further, when white cultural attitudes to grief are, rarely, examined, they too are assumed to be unitary (e.g. Kalish and Reynolds 1981). When books and therapists examine differences in styles of grieving within families, this is characteristically put down to individual differences or to gender differences, rather than to different subcultures of grief within mainline white society. As I hope to show, there are a number of cultures of grief around at present, at least two of them currently fighting each other for supremacy. I make no apology for concentrating on contemporary mainstream white cultures of mourning. Even though they affect well over 90 per cent of the population (in Britain, rather less in the USA), they have received far less scholarly scrutiny than have mourning cultures among ethnic and religious minority groups. This is partly due to the relative absence of sociological and cultural studies of bereavement in the contemporary West. Bereavement research has been dominated, on the one hand, by experts in psychology, psychiatry, therapy and counselling who concentrate on the individual, mentioning the social context only in passing, if at all. The same is true of the many books by bereaved people themselves, though they almost all include fascinating insights for readers on the look-out for cultural data. Even the growing literature on bereavement in relation to family systems is relatively silent on the influence of culture (an exception being Shapiro 1994, 1996). On the other hand, historians and anthropologists *have* researched mourning cultures, but in other places and other times.

This all gives the impression that in the contemporary West, white men and women grieve according to the dictates of a natural and inner 'grief process', a process supported or inhibited by culture but not interacting with it in any more complex way, whereas in the past and outside of the white West, grief is assumed to interact with culture in important and subtle ways. This book proceeds on the assumption that white westerners are no different from anyone else: their personal grief and the culture in which they live are intimately bound up together. To ignore this is to impoverish the understanding of those who work with bereaved people, and to impoverish sociology and cultural studies by excluding from their domain a key social phenomenon.

Most western texts on bereavement make clear distinctions between the following:

- Bereavement is the objective state of having lost someone or something.
- Grief refers to the emotions that accompany bereavement.
- Mourning is the behaviour that social groups expect following bereavement.

In this over-neat formulation, culture is often believed to influence mourning but not grief, which is deemed natural, universal and purely psychological.

In this book, I argue that culture affects grief as well as mourning, and indeed grief underlies the very constitution of society.

A framework

Where then might the sociologist start? I begin with two key ideas from Emile Durkheim, the famous French sociologist who worked a hundred years ago and who was concerned to understand the sources of human solidarity. What, Durkheim (1933, 1965) asked, holds society together? Since bereavement through death entails the rupturing of social bonds, the tearing away from society of one or more of its members, Durkheim's question is likely to prove a fruitful starting point for the sociological understanding of bereavement. What is the nature of social bonds, what happens when they are ruptured and how are ruptured bonds repaired, thus putting society back together once again? Durkheim himself (1965), along with followers such as Hertz (1960), examined the role of ritual in this regard. Although I certainly do not ignore ritual, I concur with Giddens (1991) and Seale (1998) in suggesting that, in the contemporary West, conversation – informal, official and professional – is now as important as ritual in putting the Humpty Dumpty of society back together again.

More important for the structure of the book, however, are two particular concepts that were important to Durkheim (and even more so to the later American sociologist, Talcott Parsons): integration and regulation (Durkheim 1952). Every society needs institutionalized means for integrating its members and for regulating their passions. This is particularly true of the dead and those who grieve for them. Part I of this book (Living with the dead) will look at integration, particularly the integration of the dead and those associated with them (the bereaved) into the world of the living. Part II (Policing grief) looks at regulation – how cultural norms about how they should behave and feel impact on bereaved people.

Part II looks in particular at the regulation of emotions. In the vast majority of human societies, bereavement typically affects a whole range of circumstances concerning money, inheritance and shifting social status. Modernity has succeeded in regularizing most of these. Advances in nutrition, public health and medicine mean that most people now die in old age, their children having long since left home and set up their own households. Pensions, life insurance and the welfare state mean that survivors are rarely left destitute. Our material prospects depend now on educational achievements more than on the status provided by parents or husband, so bereavement does not reduce status to the extent it once did. Yet longevity provides more years for children to get attached to parents, wives to husbands, husbands to wives, siblings to siblings. So bereavement becomes less a loss of status or of income, more the loss of a deeply personal attachment.

Typically it is not the bereaved's financial or social state but their emotional state that now dominates and requires regularizing. Typically, bereavement agencies help clients manage their emotions, and may be ill-suited to clients whose needs are practical or economic.

The Prologue provides an illustrative case study of these twin themes of integration and regulation, and can be skipped and read later if the reader wants to go straight on to the theoretical meat of the book. The introductions to each Part introduce the two themes in more detail. At the end of each of the main chapters, I provide suggestions for further reading, along with questions that may prove useful for group discussion. These questions are often geared toward practice, encouraging students to use the theory and data of the chapter to explore their own personal experiences, observations and practice.

Terminology

If I were describing the culture of grief in the nineteenth century, I would have to include mourning dress, the required periods of mourning, beliefs about reunion in the next life and so forth. Writing as I am primarily about the culture of grief at the end of the twentieth century, I have to include the panoply of professional, para-professional and voluntary services that one might term 'bereavement care', along with both expert and lay beliefs about 'the grief process', 'resolution' and so forth. Here we encounter two problems, one of terminology and the other of perspective.

'Bereavement care' is an appropriate umbrella term for a range of services: it is a term used by those who deliver it, and it (correctly) hints at the care and compassion that typically motivate it. But is there an umbrella term covering all those who provide this care? 'Bereavement carer' or (in the USA) 'caregiver' is inappropriate if we restrict it to those in a defined relation to a client, as it excludes the vast majority – friends and family – who care for bereaved people. 'Bereavement counsellor' is commonly used in the UK (for example by Danbury 1996: 21), but some of those with minimal training prefer to refer to themselves as 'bereavement volunteers', while those (including some readers of this book) who have invested years in training as counsellors may resent the use of this term by anyone who has taken only a short course in listening skills. On the whole, I tend to use the term 'bereavement worker' for all those who (paid or voluntary, full-time or part-time) specialize in bereavement care, and 'practitioner' for the professionally qualified, including doctors, nurses and teachers who find themselves with bereaved clients only from time to time.

Following Dryden *et al.* (1989), I use 'counselling' as an umbrella term to describe a particular activity engaged in by many bereavement workers and other practitioners. Bereavement workers may help with tax returns, they may pick the kids up from school, they may befriend, or they may sit and listen in a highly attentive and disciplined way to what the bereaved have to say. I refer to this latter activity as bereavement counselling, an activity undertaken by many more than those who term themselves 'counsellors'. (As a university teacher and tutor, for example, though I am not a trained counsellor, I often use basic counselling skills and in that sense I do counselling. The verb may be used more widely than the noun – just as you may teach your son to fish though you are not a trained teacher, and nurse your sick child though you are not a trained nurse.)

Even when the language is clear, there remains a problem of perspective. I write as a sociologist who, like the social historian and the social anthropologist, is trying to describe and make sense of the social world, in this case the social world that bereaved people inhabit. Bereavement counselling is now part of that world, and so it is part of the *topic* that I am describing. To analyse it and related topics, I use as *resources* the methods and perspectives of sociology, supplemented by those of history and anthropology.

Here lie the seeds of a misunderstanding. In the current climate, counselling arouses strong passions, for or against. Much writing on counselling falls into one of two categories: writings by those who see counselling as a resource to help their clients, and writings by cynics and critics who see counselling as a topic to be mocked or attacked. My book, however, falls into a third and smaller category, consisting of writings that see counselling as a topic but have no motive either to promote or attack it. The book illuminates, I hope, some hitherto neglected aspects of counselling and raises some research questions that have yet to be pursued.

Prologue

The two main themes of this book are the integration of the dead and the living, and the regulation or policing of grief. The introduction presented these themes somewhat theoretically by referring to Durkheim's sociology; now I introduce them again, but in a very different way. The Prologue comprises the transcript of a taped interview I conducted in 1997 with a competent and well-adjusted white middle-class woman in her thirties about the death of her father 21 years earlier.[1] Almost every line of Fiona's story illustrates one or both of the book's two themes. Brief interpretive sections (**highlighted**) introduce these themes.

Policing grief

Fiona's account of the immediate aftermath of her father's death is dominated by the theme of a 13-year-old girl who had her own views of how to grieve, views that she recalls were repeatedly thwarted by aunts who she felt did not respect her and did not know her father particularly well. They disapproved of her behaviour, and they disapproved of both her expression and her non-expression of emotion. For Fiona, as for most mourners, this kind of policing of her grief was primarily engaged in by fellow family members. Part II attempts to make historical and sociological sense of such experiences.

My mother died when I was 10, which would have been 1973, my father when I was 13.

And can you describe what your reaction was and other people's reaction to your reaction?

When he died, the reaction was – the way I grieved, I mean when I was first told, I didn't cry. And that put a lot of people off. And also it happened on a Saturday and I went back to school on the Monday, and even the teachers at school were surprised and didn't think I should be at school, and should have stayed at home, but I wanted to go to school, and also I had exams, and I wanted to finish the exams and people just kept saying, perhaps you should stay at home, don't go to school. But no, I wanted to go to school! And also I wanted to go to school because I knew that that's what my dad would have wanted, so it wasn't just the fact that I was being dogmatic or whatever.

Was there anybody looking after you in the immediate aftermath of the death?

Well, he was taken into hospital a couple of weeks beforehand, and I didn't want to tell anyone because I wanted to look after my sister myself – she's seven years younger than me.

So, there's just the two of you?

I have an older brother, who at the time was 28. Obviously, I rang my brother. There were just the three of us to begin with. And then when he died, I was actually staying with an aunt, in her house, that Saturday.

And did she give any idea to you as to whether you should be going to school or not?

She didn't think we should be going to school at all, no.

You wanted to go because that's what your father would have wanted?

No, I wanted to go because I wanted, I suppose, normality. And I <u>liked</u> school. I was one of those odd children that <u>loved</u> school. I wanted to be with my friends, because I thought 'I don't really know these people, and I'm feeling sad, I'm feeling lonely, and confused, all those sorts of feelings, and I want to be with people who <u>know</u> me, who understand me, I want to be with my friends.'

Who were all these other people?

Relatives. When my father was first taken into hospital, the neighbour had rung one of my other aunts and the three of them appeared on the doorstep afterwards, and I was quite cross because I'd sorted everything out, you know, I'd rung my brother, he was on his way up, he was living in Devizes at the time. [400 miles south, in England]

You were in Edinburgh?

No, in a small village outside of Edinburgh. And he was coming up, and I was fine, and everything was organized, Sarah was at school, and I was very cross when they turned up and started rushing through the house saying 'It's all your fault he's ill, look at the state of this house!!!', because you know, it was untidy, and so, yes, I was very cross. A lot of anger there as well.

My father had given up work to look after the both of us, because he didn't want me to grow up too quickly. He didn't want me to take on my mother's role, so I didn't do the housework because I was supposed to do other things, you know I was going out to play, going out with friends, doing my homework. But when he became ill, I didn't think – because I'd never been brought up to think it's my job to do the washing, or whatever.

So the house got into a bit of a tip then?

It got into a real tip, I think. We had dogs, and all sorts of things. Maybe it wasn't such a tip, but my aunts were the sort who thought everything has a place and should be in its place.

So, he died on the Saturday, and you went back to school on the Monday, and did your exams, and when was the funeral?

I think it was probably the Wednesday. That's when it all hit. I mean up until then I hadn't cried. I mean I cried when he first went into hospital, and the nurse then had said that it looks like heart failure, looks like he's not going to make it, so I cried that night, and ranted and raved a bit, and then he was getting better, and he seemed to be getting much better, then on the Saturday I was told I couldn't cry, didn't cry, and then on the Wednesday again I'd gone all through the funeral and I was so 'Oh, I haven't seen these cousins for so long' but I wanted to be involved, and I was <u>pushed</u> away <u>all</u> the time, I was told to go away and go and sit down, and you know I wasn't allowed to go in the car, I had to go with my aunts, I had to stay with my sister Sarah, you know, but I felt 'I want to be <u>involved</u> in this!'.

So what exactly were you not allowed to be involved in?

I'm trying to think . . . I just have this feeling of not being involved, of not being at the front. Thinking back, I can't remember what they were stopping me doing, I can just remember feeling '<u>I</u> want to do it! I want to be there?! What are you doing?! What are you saying?! Where are you going?!' but what it was, I can't really remember.

Were these aunts running the show, or had your brother taken over?

It was my aunts, definitely. My father's brothers' wives, most of my father's brothers had died. And also my mother's sister. It was a big family. But yes they had taken over, and I wasn't very happy!

So you were more aware of being eased out than of your father's death – that hadn't really hit you?

No, it hadn't. I don't think I'd really believed it, because on the Friday I'd seen him and he was sitting up and chatting quite normally, and I'd asked him if I could go to the local fair, it happened once a year, could I go with two of my friends, and he said yes, of course, I'll see you in the evening, Saturday evening, don't come in the afternoon, go to the fair and I'll see you in the evening. And I came home from the fair, and he'd died that morning. So I think in a way as I'd seen him chatting and being his own silly self that it didn't hit.

Did you see the body?

No.

Was that your choice?

No, we weren't allowed. Other people saw it, which is why I was very cross . . . There are certain traditions in our family, apparently – the females don't go to the graveside, apart from the wife or maybe the mother, but all other females go back to the house. But I don't know whether that's a family or a cultural thing.

Did you want to go to the grave?

Yes (emphatically). Very much so. I mean that was the bit when I broke. I'd gone all through the service, and it wasn't <u>real</u>, you know, my brother was sitting in the front pew (in church) and he was kneeling throughout the whole of the service, and he just had his hand on the coffin, and I remember thinking 'What's he doing?! Why's he doing that?' and then the coffin was carried out and everyone was crying and I was just looking round and thinking 'What's going on? What's going on?' and I think then as it went into the hearse, as the doors were closing, I just suddenly thought 'My dad's in there! And I haven't seen him!!' you know, and I got very agitated then, and er, I said 'I want to come, I want to come' and they said 'No you can't. We've spoken, and you're <u>not</u> going to the graveside. You can go home with Aunt Helen.' 'I want to go! I want to go!' 'No, you can't.' And then what <u>really</u> did it was my cousin who's female, Susan, went to the grave as the representative of the school. So she was allowed to go, she had her school uniform on as the representative of the school. And that was it – wafff! And that was when I cried. And the rest of the afternoon is just a complete blank. I can remember at my aunt's house the local doctor sitting with me, saying 'Are you all right?', so . . . ?!

Clearly then your reaction was a mixture of anger at all these people as well as the loss of your dad?

I think it was mostly anger, I think the loss didn't hit me at all then. It was anger, you know 'Why am I being kept out?' Maybe it's the little princess syndrome. I was always there, I was always told everything, and now I'm not important any more. I remember anger, the strongest feeling I remember up until the day of the funeral, anger at everything and everyone, and having to move out of the house and having to stay with my aunts.

When did you move out of the house?

I think Sunday. My brother, I don't think he wanted to stay in the house any more, after dad had died, so he moved us all out. Then we stayed with my aunt a short while.

So if you wanted to go back to school because that's where your friends were, presumably you'd want to be at home for the same reason – that's where the familiar things are?

Yes, I did, but it was too painful for my brother to stay, and he obviously couldn't leave a 13-year-old and a 6-year-old on their own, but I wanted to be in my <u>own</u> bed in my <u>own</u> room.

You seem a little more forgiving of your brother?

Yes, I was <u>very</u> forgiving of him because he was also quite young, 28, I think it swept over him. He was a single man whose life was suddenly turned upside down. It would never be the same again. He now had two girls to be responsible for.

So you then stayed with your aunts? How did things go then in terms of how people expected you to be?

Well, apparently I didn't do <u>anything</u> they expected me to do, and I caused problems. My father died in the April, and by the end of May, I was asked to leave. So my brother had to go to court, because he was in the army, so he could get somewhere to live for us, so we had to become a ward of the court, to him, so he could go back to the army to get somewhere to live. Meanwhile, till October, I stayed with a cousin and her family, so I could stay on at the school till the end of the year. It was better, but she still had this 'You're a spoiled little brat, behave yourself! It's been months now, you shouldn't still be behaving like this.' I don't know what she meant, I was just being me!

And I think a lot of people had a problem with my attitude. My father had always brought us up to speak our mind, whereas my mother's brother's family was always very much 'Children should be seen and not heard'. And also the girls in the house should do all the housework! You know, home-work comes second! Whereas at home, homework was first and, you know, I had chores, but they came second.

How well did your aunt and your cousin know your father?

This is where it begins to get tough. Not very well at all. There had been a big row many years before I was born. We were Catholic, but my uncle is an Orangeman, and there was a lot of bad feeling between him and my father. The uncle with whom I was staying . . . I think the anger came from this. She hadn't set foot in the house for many, many years, even before my mother died, then suddenly she was walking in the door without even knocking on it. And I apparently told her that 'Everything was under control and that she could leave'!!! I mean she kept this for many years apparently, it wasn't until my sister's wedding in the late 1980s that she told of being turned out of the house by a 13-year-old. Yes, I wasn't happy, and the cousins weren't happy to have me there, and it was very difficult. And again, it was very difficult because I should have cried on the first day, and that upset her, because she then didn't know how to deal with me, and then because I was in such a state <u>afterwards</u>, that wasn't right either. And going back to school, 'Why should I go back to school?' and you know, people didn't know how to react to me, maybe. That's me looking back; when it was happening, it was just happening. Maybe they wanted to comfort me, but I wasn't going to be comforted! I had <u>exams</u> to do.

Did you cry a lot in the weeks and months afterwards?

I did, for a long, long time afterwards, it was just as if it wouldn't stop. Even now, I have tissues here! I was never a crying child, and it was almost as if when my father died, I'd cry at anything, TV programmes, you name it. Ever since!

Continuing the bond

Fiona now goes on to talk about the ongoing place of her father in her life. She and her young sister had to move 400 miles to the south of England to the bare quarters given to her brother by the army, with none of her old familiar possessions; this left only her sister as a link with the childhood she had known, the only tangible link with her father. Her sister experiences her father, but does not make a habit of speaking to him. Fiona does not have such a direct experience, but chooses to maintain the bond with her father by regularly speaking to him. Such phenomena are discussed in Chapter 3, 'Private bonds'. Other family members want her to forget her father and what he stood for, as discussed in Chapter 2.

So you moved down to England in October?

Yes, that's where nightmare phase two began! It was just completely different from anything I'd ever known. All the furniture had been sold because we girls were expected to stay with relatives. All the books were got rid of because my aunts didn't have many books whereas we had loads . . . I'd always been expected to contribute, you know, my father would always say 'what do you think?', 'what shall we do?', even simple things like 'what shall we have for tea tonight?', I was <u>always</u> being asked for my opinion, and suddenly I was put into this situation where decisions were being made <u>for</u> me and I am still cross that the toys, the furniture, everything, <u>my</u> things, had gone. Okay, fair enough, they wanted to get rid of the memories of mum and dad, but not my things! . . . And also they didn't agree with the way my father was bringing us up, so I was constantly being told 'You may have got away with that at <u>home</u>, with your <u>father</u>, but not here.' I was constantly being told that I'd been wrapped up in cotton wool, that no-one was allowed to say anything against me, and I was a little princess – but I wasn't really.

So you had to fit into the regime of their family. How did your brother bring you up?

He didn't cope too well. He had a lot of problems I think. He wasn't single any more, but he wasn't married either. I think he took my parents' death very hard. He didn't allow any photographs, we couldn't talk about him. He just got too upset.

So your father didn't really have a presence in the household then?

No, there were no photographs of him or us. They were all in a box, sealed. A totally alien place to be.

You felt that at the time?

Oh yes.

What did you feel?

Devastated, completely devastated. Just, where do I belong? What is this place, this bare, empty shell? (Describes garish military furnishings of the flat). And the complete isolation was hard . . .

Was your sister the one link with the past, then?

Yes, she was the constant. It was then that I became, I suppose, the mother. She was mine, she was the link . . .

Do you remember ways in which you tried to keep your father's memory alive in this very alien situation?

Talking to him. That was the only thing I could do, talk to him.

Out loud, or quietly?

Quietly. In my head!

Can you remember what sort of things you said to him?

Yea, but I'd probably get upset if I told you.

Did your sister talk to him as well?

No, she didn't. Because I can remember telling her once to talk to him, because she was getting upset, and she said 'Don't be silly. He's dead.' What she actually said was 'He told me he was dead when he came to visit me.' And I went cold! And she said 'On the second night that we moved in, I woke up and daddy was sitting on the end of my bed, and I said 'Why are you here?' and he said 'Well, I'm dead. But I still love you, and I'm still looking after you' and I went back to sleep.' She said 'There's no point in talking to him, because he's dead.'

Apart from your sister, did you tell anybody else that you talked to your father?

No, not until today . . . I talked to him out loud when I was giving birth! That upset my husband, because I was calling for my <u>father</u>. I can remember wanting him. My experience of a physical thing came then after the birth, you know I said my sister had a physical thing, but I never did. I used to lie in bed and pretend that he was holding my hand, but I <u>knew</u> that I was pretending. I didn't feel anything. But after the birth of my first child, I can remember going back, it was quite a traumatic birth, and I recall lying there, completely exhausted, and being upset wishing mum and dad could see her, and as I thought it, I felt, two hands, one here and one here, on my wrists, and my pain seemed to go, and I thought – wow – they've seen her, and this is their way of telling me. And I woke up in the morning, and thought don't be silly, it's the drugs, and I told my husband and said it was obviously the way you were holding my hand, and he said, no, we weren't holding your hand, we were holding you under the arm and your leg. No one touched your hand! I'm still a bit sceptical that it may have been the drugs . . . It was as though, suddenly in my head, 'we've seen her'. But whether that's me, or really was them, I don't know. It was a very traumatic birth.

Talking about the dead

Chapter 4 argues that one of the main ways in which the dead are kept alive is in everyday conversation among the living. Fiona consciously attempts to keep the memory of her father alive, even in her children who never met him but now know him through her.

I'm told one great thing about the first baby is being able to show your own parents.

Yes, that was the hardest thing, not being able to . . . I spoke to her all the time about her grandad and her grandma, from day one, I'd say 'Oh your grandad would think you're beautiful!' and while feeding her I used to tell her stories that dad used to tell me and the things that we used to do together. I mean all the time I'd talk to her – this was a 2-day-old baby!

Do you still do it?

I still do it yes.

Does that make it easier in a way now that you have someone you can talk to about your dad?

Um, I think so, yes I think it does, and I think it's helped my brother. The sealed box I told you about is no longer sealed, the box with all the photographs. One of the girls had a project to do about the Second World War, and my father wrote a diary, and my brother actually got this diary out and photocopied it so she could take it to school. There was his medals, and his shaving mirror. And my brother finds it different now he can talk to my girls about their grandad, where for so many years he couldn't even say his name.

So your dad has a kind of conversational presence in your household now because of your children?

Yes.

Was he in the conversation between you and your husband before the children came along?

Um, yes, yes. I'd say, 'Oh, dad and I used to do this' or if, say Christmas traditions, I'd say 'Well, in <u>my</u> household!', because his family didn't have traditions, didn't have things like that.

So before you got married? Do you need marriage and family for your dad to be part of the conversation?

I talked to my friends about him, eventually, when I was in the sixth form. It started with one of my friends at school at Devizes saying 'You're going to <u>hate</u> me for saying this, but I'm glad that your dad died, because if he hadn't I'd never have met you' and that was it then, we started talking about him. And another friend of mine whose father used to hit them, and had an affair in the end, she used to say 'You are actually lucky you had a good childhood, you have happy memories of when you were little, even though you don't have it now. I haven't, all I have is hatred' so we could then talk about things.

So he disappeared from actual conversations with other people for a few years, but he was there in your memory and in your conversations with him. And only later did he become a more regular part of the conversation. Do you feel that he's therefore more with you now than when you were, say, 15 or 16?

Oh, no (immediately and definitely), he was always with me quite strongly. I've always had a strong feeling. No, I didn't feel 'At last, I can talk to someone about him', it was just a natural progression. I would have talked to him, to anyone who would have listened. It's just not what 14- or 15-year-olds talk about . . .

Professional help

Fiona goes on to recall her experiences of counselling by a well-meaning doctor who was concerned that Fiona, now in her late teens, was suffering from unresolved grief. She experiences the doctor as applying a model of grief that did not fit her own self-understanding, and just added further to her problems. According to Fiona, he mistakenly concentrates on grief having to run its natural course, and has difficulty understanding the problems created by her aunts' policing activities; further, he assumes that the primary loss of her father must be more traumatic than the secondary losses that followed from it – loss of home and loss of familiar surroundings. All these assumptions Fiona feels were incorrect. Her experience of the doctor illustrates that professionals may have difficulty in letting go of their pre-conceived notions of grief and in really listening to the client. The doctor's counselling skills may not have been the best in the world, but may well be typical of the kind of professional help that the average bereaved person actually receives. (In the UK, general practitioners are the most likely professional for bereaved people to approach in the first instance.)

Earlier Fiona had tried to join her father by committing suicide, and here her religious beliefs as a Catholic seem important as she tries to work out the practicalities of this: not only the practicalities of how to commit suicide, but also how to ensure their paths will actually meet after her death. We see here a teenage girl caught between the world of the dead (represented by trying to rejoin her father) and the world of the living (represented by a professional who was not on the same wavelength). Doubtless Fiona was perceived as a somewhat uncooperative client. Fortunately for her, she eventually found another professional – a priest – who provided an account of her problems that she could embrace.

These issues of the role of expert theories of grief, how they are applied by professionals, and how bereaved people seek out individuals and groups with stories that match their own are explored in Chapters 6, 9 and 11. The role of religion is touched on in Chapter 1, especially the greater ability of Catholicism (compared with Protestantism) to articulate relations between the living and the dead. This section raises once again Fiona's desire to keep her father alive in the conversation (Chapter 4) and in the material artefacts (Chapter 3) of her own family life.

You mentioned a GP [family doctor] who thought you had arrested grief or something?

Yes, that was in Devizes.

What happened there?

I don't know. Going back to your question about what I said to my father, I think I almost went into a fantasy world. After my mock A levels [high school exams taken around age 18], I decided I couldn't do it, I didn't even want to go out any more at night, I got very frightened. I kept thinking everyone's talking about me, I don't want to be here any more, and I was really getting into a bit of a state, wouldn't go to school, so my brother said 'Maybe you'd better go and see the doctor', so we went along, my brother came with me, and the doctor said 'you've lost your parents?' and my brother said 'Yes, she took it very hard' and that was it, he said 'Oh yes, right, I think the problem is you need to complete your grief process, you haven't grieved properly, and you're still grieving, and we need to sort out those issues before we can get you back on track'.

What did you think about that?

I thought it was a load of nonsense! I thought 'What, grief? What do you mean? What are you talking about?' And he gave me valium, and I didn't think any more about it. It was intended to get me back to school and back to work.

And what did you think was going on?

I think maybe it was just – looking back, that is – because my brother wasn't married he wasn't entitled to this flat. At 18 I was no longer a ward of court, and had to be <u>out</u>. Two or three days after my eighteenth birthday. That was worrying me. Where was I going to stay, where was I going to live? And the stress of the exams. And we'd lost our Chemistry teacher, so I had to change exam subjects, so I think that with all that pressure, all that stress, I just caved in for a little while. I don't think it had anything to do with the grief at all . . .

But I did feel guilty about being angry at my dad for leaving me, and for the move to Devizes. 'Why did you leave me?! Why didn't you know this was going to happen? Why didn't you go to the doctor? You were the adult, you were the grown up! <u>You</u> should have gone to the doctor.' There was anger that he'd gone to be with my mother (my aunts said he'd never last long after her death). He missed her so much, he talked about her openly, he had a very hard time. He talked about how much he loved her, how much he missed her.

Did you talk to other people about this, or was this more the conversations you had with your father?

Yes, this was all internal.

So after she died, he talked about how much he missed her, and that was the sort of conversation you were used to, so the style of grieving you had to engage in after your father died was completely different?

Yes. There was no one to talk to, I mean people would get upset and then they'd stop talking and go away, and I'd think 'What's wrong with these grown-ups? Grown-ups are supposed to cry and hug you! What's wrong with them? Why are they trying to stop themselves crying? It's normal to rant and rave and shout!'

When you were able to talk about your father, did that feel good?

Yes . . . My father always said, 'No-one ever dies as long as someone still remembers them, so you must always remember your family, your great grandparents, your grandparents, you must always talk about it, tell your children. I suppose the guilt comes in here that I can't remember all the things he told me about his parents. I feel guilty, and can't keep it alive for the girls. That's quite strongly instilled in me. So I talk about my father and my mother, and we've got pictures of them in the house as well, so they're alive, their memory's alive, and there are things to hand down. Although a lot of things went, there are my mother's wedding rings, there are three, so each of us has one, and they'll be passed down . . .

What did you believe about where your father was?

That was a tough one for me, a very tough one. My father lost his faith after my mother died, but we still went to church, you know, he sent us, and the night he was taken into hospital I have never prayed so hard! All night. So when he died, I thought, you know, obviously no God, nobody here. So I don't know where I thought he went, but because I wanted to follow him, and I had a few attempts, there was also the feeling of – this is maybe Catholic indoctrination – that if he has gone to heaven, I think I was worried that if he had died not knowing God, you know, not believing, then that would mean he'd be in purgatory, so I was thinking, I've got to pray so hard so he gets out of there quickly! But at the same time, not really believing, 'cos if there was such a thing it wouldn't have happened. I had quite a few suicide attempts and I think at the back of my mind, what was stopping me was, well 'It's a sin, and if I take my own life, I won't go to heaven, and if he has gone to heaven, then I won't be with him anyway!' But I was just very bad at it anyway! But I just wanted to be with him, I didn't want to be left behind. So, I suppose, I was hoping he would be in heaven, that he had made his peace. That came from my aunts, that didn't come from the priest. The priest was no comfort to me at all. It was the aunts who went on about purgatory, and we all had to pray for him, and that made it worse, that made it really, really tough. But since then, I've spoken to other priests, about purgatory, about beliefs and things.

Do you think he might have got to heaven a bit quicker then?

I think, yea, I think he is, I think he did.

How did people respond to your suicide attempts?

That was because, you know, I hadn't accepted the death properly. That was what the hospital said. I'm actually quite vague on the time-scale. The Scotland one was just shortly after his death and I was standing over this little bridge, and thinking 'I want to be with you' but then I looked down and 'But what if I drown!!' I could do it if I could convince myself I'd kill myself on the way down with the impact, but I was terrified I was going to drown! And I thought the bridge might not be high enough. And then I thought it's a sin and I'd go straight to hell, and not find my dad because he'll be in purgatory.

All the suicide attempts were seen as related to my father's death, that I needed to talk about it. And then I was saying 'Well, I don't want to talk about it to you. Don't want to talk about it <u>now</u>, thank you very much!' I had a counsellor who came to the house, and I wouldn't talk to her either. I was very awkward, I think! The person I did talk to was my friend, and I thought 'No, I don't need these counsellors anyway, I'll talk to my friend.' And what she did was take me back to the church, and then I spoke to a priest, who's become a very close friend, and he did the trick. He said 'It's not that you're not grieving properly, it's not that you haven't said goodbye properly. It's more to do with the fact that you were wrenched away from your family, from everything that you knew – a totally different way of life, a big school. It's the pressure of having to find somewhere to live at your age, worrying who's going to look after Sarah, worry about your brother, it's much more to do with that than with the fact that you've lost your father.' I thought, 'Ha, knew it!' No, I didn't really.

Do you think the counsellor would have done better without a pre-definition of what was wrong?

Yes, even the GP, I thought 'Why are people talking about his death? This has got nothing to do with that. Yes, he's dead, I miss him, I want him back, I want to be with him, but why are they talking about <u>grieving</u>?' That's the word they kept on using, and I didn't know what they were trying to get me to do. As far as I was concerned, I had grieved, I was still grieving, I am still grieving, I don't think it's a process that has a beginning, a middle and an end. You know, I think people have an individual way of grieving. My brother was totally different, he just went completely insular, didn't want to know, didn't want to talk. I remember my father saying 'I wish he'd talk to me, I wish he'd say how he's feeling.'. . . At the time I was completely confused by all this, what I should be doing, how I should be feeling. 'How did I feel when?' 'How do you think I felt?! Stupid question!!' And 'What upset you the most?' 'Well, it was my aunts!' They said, 'No, no, no, you know, more personal than that, what upset you most about the loss of your father?' 'No, no, my aunts! You're not listening to me, you don't understand.' That was an incredible feeling. That was both the doctor and the counsellor.

Becoming an ancestor

In the final section, Fiona gives further instances of how as a youngster, and now as a mother, she continues to practise modes of behaviour she had learned from her father. Her father lives on, not just in memory, not just in conversation, but in behavioural patterns that he initiated and that Fiona chooses to perpetuate. As a teenager, she had to struggle against her aunt who had a different view of parenting from her father, but as a mother she can embrace his mode of parenting as she brings up her own children. She ends by describing the steps she is currently taking to ensure that her own children do not have to face the obstacles living with their ancestors that she, Fiona, had to overcome. Whereas psychologists have analysed how the dead can be internalized within the psyche of the survivor, Fiona illustrates the theme of Part I, namely that the dead can live on in more public ways, actually influencing social behaviour, even in a secular society in which languages for articulating such roles for the dead have withered.

My aunt wouldn't let me go to football matches any more, even though my father's friends said they'd still take me, you know my father used to take me every Saturday – I'd go to watch Hibs play. And she wouldn't let me go. So that was that – big argument! I did go actually, on a couple of occasions. On a few Saturdays, I actually went across to the pub where they got on the coach and I'd say 'She said it was all right today, I can come' and I'd told her I'd gone off to play with friends, but I was actually going to watch the football, and I'd be dreading it'd be on TV that night. But she never found out! . . . I'd think 'Please dad come back! This isn't right – I want to go to the football!'. . .

   After my mother's death, my aunts wanted my father to go back to work, and they were going to look after us and he said 'No way! I'm bringing you up my way. I'm not having anyone else bring you up.' Which I think has stayed with me. Even at that age, I remember thinking 'No, I'm not going to change, I'm going to be like this, the way my father wanted to be, this is the way I'm going to be.' And even with my girls now, I think I base how I bring them up on the way he brought me up, and the things he told me are exactly what I'm telling them. Because I think it was right. But I know that it isolated them from the rest of the family, because they didn't agree.

I'm struck by how much you remember in detail.

It's all I had, I had nothing else, nothing to look at, nothing to hold, nothing to touch, so in my mind every night, I'd hear the stories, I'd say 'Dad, tell me about when . . .' and then I'd listen to the stories, I could hear his voice. What worries me as I get older is how much of that memory is the real actual event, and how much is me wanting, or adding bits to it? That's what worries me . . .

When Alison was quite young, from about two, I started thinking about my mother, 'I don't know anything about her, I don't know her favourite colour, favourite food.' So I thought 'If anything happens to me, I don't want my girls to have the same kind of, you know, missing part of their family' so I started writing things down, things like, thoughts on your birth, this is how I felt. It's not a diary, it's just a sheet of paper which I keep on adding to . . . The girls don't know about it, it's just if anything happens to me.

Note

1 The interview was intended as neither therapy nor research. I encountered Fiona in the course of my work as an academic, and a chance conversation indicated that her experience of bereavement illustrated the major themes of this book. She responded positively to my request to conduct an interview in order to gather illustrative material. At the time of the interview, she had not read any of my writings on bereavement. I have deleted a modest amount of extraneous material from the transcript (indicated by . . .). Fiona read the transcript, slightly revised it and chose pseudonyms for herself and her family.

The interview is entirely retrospective, covering events up to 21 years ago. I make no claim that the interview documents how Fiona actually felt then. Rather it documents how she perceives and remembers those events and feelings now, and how she talked about them – with considerable passion and clarity – in a taped interview.

PART I

Living with the dead

Introduction to Part I

Lizzie, the 9-year-old daughter of Juno and older sister of Nancy, is dead. Juno says, I don't know what I'd do if (Nancy) wasn't here. If I hadn't had her I would have killed myself. I wanted to die to see where (Lizzie) was. To see someone was looking after her. I wanted to go for five minutes but I wanted to come back. Nancy is my link to keep me on earth.

(Cline 1996: 190)

Juno here describes the situation of many bereaved people, caught between the world of the living and the world of the dead. Somehow, they must traverse this boundary. This can be a strange experience for them, and disturbing for their friends and relations. The more the bereaved live with the dead, the more they are marginalized by a historically Protestant and now largely secular society that has difficulty articulating such relationships; the more they live with the living, the worse they feel about abandoning the dead. Both the dead and the bereaved must somehow find a place in, and be integrated into, society.

This existence in no man's land, betwixt and between two realities, one past, one present, is not, psychologically speaking, unique to bereavement through death. On grieving the demise of a love affair, the abandoned lover's thoughts are constantly with the lost one, yet s/he must somehow live in the ongoing everyday world, a world that may now seem unreal or meaningless. The unemployed man may continue to get up at six every morning, even though there is no job to go to. Some days after a mountaineering accident, I returned home to find that the everyday world of the mortgage and shopping and work seemed less real than the life-and-death drama of a few days before. Returnees from battle have had similar experiences, finding it hard to reintegrate back into their families and into civilian life. Such experiences of dissociation are not unusual.

Bereavement through death, however, is inevitably social as well as psychological: the integration of the past (the dead) into the present must be negotiated not just within the head of the individual mourner, but within society itself. If society cannot integrate its dead, then it loses touch with its past, it has no history. This is most clear in the remembrance rituals following war or civil war (Chapter 2), but it is also true of peacetime deaths. How bereaved people integrate the dead into their own lives is central to how society itself perpetuates itself, for if the dead are not integrated then society disconnects from its own past and ultimately from itself. Bereavement and history are much more closely intertwined than conventional disciplinary boundaries might imply. It is this long-term impact of bereavement that differentiates bereavement in humans from bereavement in other animals, for they are not eternally bound to the past through personal and cultural history (Kaplan 1995: 16–17) – or if they are, it is through learned behaviour rather than through belief systems and conscious memory. As Cox and Gilbert put it (1986: ix), 'Whatever we do with the dead they will not go away . . . We have no option but to learn to live with them.'

Learning to live with the dead is something that even those who never met them may have to deal with, even if it is by banishing them. One little boy's mother died when he was two and his father remarried four years later. The stepmother was so jealous of the father's relationship with the boy's mother that she would not allow any mention of the little boy's past or of his mother. It has been said that in any remarriage (whether through death or divorce) there are three people (Moss and Moss 1996), but the new partner may refuse to acknowledge this. The new partners must negotiate a place for the dead in the new marriage, or ban the dead from the new marriage, or allow the dead to dominate and haunt the present. Finding an appropriate place for the dead is, therefore, not just for the *individual* mourner, as so many texts (e.g. Worden 1991) imply, but may be a task with which non-mourners also have to deal.

This example also makes us ask whether Cox and Gilbert are right. Maybe it is possible to leave the dead behind? Certainly many people in contemporary western cultures want to do this, while in a number of other cultures (such as the Apache) it is forbidden to speak the names of the dead (Rosenblatt *et al.* 1976: ch.4). The question of how Anglo/American culture incorporates the dead into everyday conversation is discussed at length in Chapters 4 and 5.

We have, then, the possibility of the dead being under-integrated into society, and some would suggest this is the case in Britain and the USA today. A society in love with youth, progress and the future will turn its back on its ancestors, lose touch with its past, and abandon traditional rituals of mourning. But even the USA has not gone entirely down this road. With immigrant forebears who left their ancestors behind in Europe or Asia, some Americans enthusiastically set about tracing their roots. But on the whole, it is modern, forward looking countries that have the most difficulty integrating the dead, unless they be the famous dead.

The other extreme possibility is of the dead being over-integrated. This is likely to occur in static societies in which elders and ancestors control everyday life. Again, in practice, it may be more complex. According to Bloch (1971), the Merina of Madagascar live in two worlds: the everyday world and the symbolic, ritual world of the ancestors. Involvement with the ancestors frees the Merina to tackle the changing world of contemporary Madagascar, an analysis that is congruent with Marris's (1974) view that humans need to retain some contact with what they have lost if they are to remain secure enough to face the challenge of change.

By rupturing human bonds, death threatens social solidarity; by affirming social bonds, the rituals of mourning reconstitute society. Such is the received wisdom of Durkheimian-influenced social anthropology (Huntington and Metcalf 1979; Bloch and Parry 1982). Our mortal human condition that threatens social solidarity is transformed into the very source of solidarity; death tears apart and yet the repair work creates society. As Peter Berger, one of the very few sociologists to integrate mortality into his theory of society, put it (1969: 52) 'Every human society is, in the last resort, men banded together in the face of death.' No death, and there would be less need to band together. I think of a friend who lost his father when he was 15-years-old; for the next three weeks, his mother, his sisters and he slept in the same room, reflecting what may be a basic human instinct for survivors to cling together. When Diana, Princess of Wales died in 1997, leaving behind 15- and 12-year-old sons, mothers in their thousands swept up their children and travelled up to London to lay flowers at Kensington Palace, affirming their own familial solidarity in defiance of the death that had ruptured one symbolic family (Walter 1999b). At the global level, Diana's funeral united people world-wide into the biggest television audience of all time. Warner (1959: 248) has analysed Memorial Day ceremonies in the USA in similar terms.

Over two hundred years ago, as Britain evolved from a religious society, in which the fear of hell induced morality, to a more individualistic and commercial society, Adam Smith pondered what now would provide the shared morality without which society would fall apart. Might it be the fellow feeling that is expressed following bereavement? Might sympathy be one root of solidarity (Smith 1759/1976; Schor 1994)? This foreshadows Durkheim: involvement in groups generates sentiments and mutual sentiment generates social solidarity. My message to sociologists is that we should not forget the insight of Smith, Durkheim and the anthropologists that how a society re-forms itself after a death may be one key to understanding social solidarity. The sociology of death and loss may turn out to be not a minor and rather esoteric specialism, but central to the question of how modern societies hold together.

Yet while some rituals incorporate the dead, others banish them (Bauman 1992). Removing the body to the undertakers, isolating mourners from ongoing social life for a specified period, leaving food by the grave to ensure that the dead are well fed and need not return to haunt the living – all these rituals serve to banish the dead. Certainly some mourning rituals can serve to integrate the dead into society and thus integrate society; but other rituals serve to keep the dead away and thus prevent the living from getting so bogged down in thoughts of death that the will to live is undermined. Modern societies that keep the dying, the dead and the grieving at arm's length are by no means unique, nor even particularly extreme.[1] Just as the bereaved individual has to find a place somewhere between life and death, so too do societies. In each case, ritual (Davies 1997) and conversation (Walter 1996b; Seale 1998) are primary vehicles by means of which this place is arrived at.

That place is not static, however. Stroebe and Schut (1999), looking at the psychology of grieving individuals, have developed a 'dual process model' in which the mourner oscillates between experiencing the emotional pain of grief and attending to the practical and possibly radically new tasks of living. In the framework I have outlined above, we may re-cast this as oscillation between the dead and the living and I suggest that it is not only individuals but also entire societies that can oscillate between death and life. Just as there is no predicting how an individual mourner will oscillate, so too with societies. It *is* possible, however, to look back and trace the history of oscillation, which is what Chapters 1 and 2 will sketch for a number of societies. Chapters 3, 4 and 5 will then look in more detail at how bonds with the dead are constructed, maintained and challenged in contemporary western societies, while Chapter 6 discusses how all this relates to traditional theories of grief.

Note

1 For critiques of the idea of modern society being 'death denying', see Kellehear (1983), Walter (1991a), and Seale (1998: ch. 3).

1 Other places, other times

The notion of a 'traditional' society is fraught with difficulties. Pre-modern and non-western societies are highly varied and it is impossible to generalize. Yet, both sociologists and would-be reformers of the modern way of death have often posited happy dying in a communal traditional society as a way of pointing up the failures of contemporary dying and grieving. They imply that there is a 'natural' way of dying and grieving which has been messed up by industrialization/secularization/individualism/urbanization (take your pick), and if only we would rediscover and tune in to what we intuitively know to be natural then we can once more die and grieve contentedly. Such misuse of history has been criticized by Walter (1995) and by Floersch and Longhofer (1997), and I have no desire here to romanticize the past. The anthropological and historical evidence gives little ground to hope that traditional funeral rituals *necessarily* assisted individuals through grief, nor that the needs of the bereaved explain the existence of funeral and mourning rituals (Huntington and Metcalf 1979: 44; Gittings 1984). Rituals may help the individual mourner; they may not.

There are good reasons, however, for surveying the evidence in non-modern societies. Whereas bereavement research in the contemporary West has focused on the individual's emotions and adjustment to new roles and identities, anthropological studies of traditional societies have focused instead on public rituals and on the role of the dead. Historical studies of death in the Middle Ages in Europe have likewise examined religion and relationships between the living and the dead. We may therefore learn much about such matters by looking at studies of other cultures and other times.

Dialogues with the dead

In many non-western societies, the bond between living and dead is not perceived as existing solely, if at all, within the head of the bereaved individual. There are two reasons why this may be hard for the Western reader to grasp. One is that we modern westerners have rather few ways of talking together about the dead; memories of the dead have become largely private, a matter of the psychology of grief more than of how a community remembers itself. The second is that, since Freud, bereavement theory has effectively abolished the dead, seeing the changes that follow death as occurring solely within the psyche of the bereaved individual or at most within family dynamics. The Sora of eastern India, by contrast, analyse not the bereaved, but the dead, who in turn communicate with the living. At times, the dead nurture their living descendants, at other times inflict upon them the very illnesses from which they died. Dialogues with the dead occur not in the head of the bereaved person, but through a shaman in ritual trance (Vitebsky 1993). Such ritual dialogues can occur within the modern West, notably through Catholic prayers for the dead and through Spiritualist mediums, but such dialogues are generally regarded as somewhat marginal to everyday life and at odds with the dominant materialist and scientific world-view.

In societies where relationships with the dead are accepted, they are typically articulated through religion. Durkheim's student Robert Hertz (1960, first published 1907) argued that rites which involve the corpse and the mourners cannot be separated from rites that involve the soul. Thus in rural Greece (Danforth 1982), for five years after the funeral the body lies in a splendid marble grave. Each evening, the widow or closest female relative comes to tend the grave, to pray for the dead person, to remember; at their nightly vigil the women talk with each other and swap stories. At the end of five years they dig up the grave and inspect the bones, a traumatic business for the chief mourner as she sees before her eyes what her husband, child or parent has been reduced to. If the bones are white and clean, the women take this to mean that the soul is now cleansed of its sins and is in paradise. They collect the bones and place them in the communal village ossuary, and the mason can re-use the marble for the next burial. If the bones are not clean, they are placed back in the grave, prayer is multiplied, and another year or two elapses before the women try again.

Following Hertz, Danforth suggests that what happens over time to the corpse, soul and mourners is all of a piece.

- The corpse is decaying. Its putrid flesh is consumed by the earth, until after a few years only clean bones are left. At this point the bones lose their individual identity as they are tossed into the ossuary and become the unidentifiable bones of ancestors.

- The individual soul is being purified, aided by the prayers of the living, so that it can join the company in paradise.
- The mourner is grieving the loss of husband, child or parent. This pain is unique to her but, once the ritual mourning is over, the deceased moves from being uniquely grieved by one person to being one of the village ancestors.

This multifaceted work is typically seen by the participants not as grief work but as spiritual work (du Boulay 1990). It makes sense to them only in terms of assisting the deceased soul in its passage away from this world and into the next and without this religious perspective the ritual would collapse. Following Geertz (1973), Danforth argues that the religious perspective offers a 'really real' reality beyond the objective reality of everyday life.

> It is in the context of this religious perspective, in the language of religious rituals and funeral laments, that the conversation between the living and the dead is carried on. Within this perspective the souls of the dead exist and have needs that are met by the daily visits of women to the graveyard. This is the reality generated by religious ritual and validated by religious belief.
>
> (Danforth 1982: 139)

The women are aware of the tension between these two realities, sometimes muttering to themselves that all the work they do cleaning and tidying the grave does not help the soul at all: 'It's all useless. It's all for nothing.' (Danforth 1982: 140). Nor is there any guarantee that this spiritual work eases their grief. After all, bereaved Greek men seem to cope quite nicely without any of this time-consuming ritual, meeting as usual with their mates in the coffee shop. The religious perspective is the basis of dialogues with the dead in Japan (Yamamoto et al. 1969), Tibetan Buddhism (Goss and Klass 1997), Judaism (Ribner 1998), medieval Europe (Geary 1994), and many other cultures (Parkes et al. 1997). It is not always clear to what extent the members of these cultures share the doubts of the Greek women as to the efficacy of their spiritual labours. But we may expect that, in a more secular modern West in which the religious perspective is seen to reflect a personal choice rather than a real reality (Berger 1969), dialogues with the dead are likely to become private and even secret. This is indeed what we find in Chapter 3.

We should not assume that in those societies that acknowledge the role of the dead everyone can become an ancestor, or that becoming an ancestor has to do with the needs of the bereaved. Among the Tallensi of Ghana, ancestors comprise only those who in life held authority – which they continue to wield after death. Appeal to their authority in turn legitimates that exercised by the living (Fortes 1965):

It is not the whole person but only the jural status as someone vested with authority and responsibility that is transmitted into ancestorhood. This explains why beliefs about the mode of existence of ancestor spirits are usually very vague. Those who venerate ancestors are generally unable to say very much about what form they take, where they are or what kind of existence they lead. They are unconcerned about such things . . . Neither does veneration of ancestors depend at all upon what actual relations between the deceased and the descendant(s) were like when the former was alive. It has nothing at all to do with individual feelings.

(Hamilton 1998: 21)

For the Tallensi, ancestors have more to do with legitimating the authority system than with bereavement or personal attachment to the dead. Ancestors in China and Japan seem generally less authoritative, less interfering and less punitive than African ancestors. This may be because in China and Japan, authority is not vested wholly in senior kinsmen, but is split between them and state and local bureaucracies (Wolf 1974).

The banned dead

While many societies expect the living to engage in ritualized dialogues with the dead, some others ban any discourse with the dead or may not allow the name of the dead person to be mentioned. The Hopi Indians of Arizona do not like the idea of death and are afraid of the newly dead. Though weeping may be unavoidable, it is not encouraged and should be done alone, outside the village where nobody can see. The Hopi express no desire to recall the memory of the dead and though they are not required to destroy the deceased's property they do not wish to be reminded of them – photographs are particularly offensive (Mandelbaum 1959). Certain Apache groups, by contrast, vigorously mourn the newly dead, but then proceed to banish all trace of them. Opler (1936) relates this to the ambivalence that Apaches feel about their relatives, which extends to a fear of the relative's ghost. Rosenblatt et al. (1976: ch.4) have identified a number of cultures that require similar kinds of tie-breaking.

Is this similar to those contemporary Americans and Britons who quickly sell the deceased's possessions, move house and decline to speak of the dead? Not necessarily. Many traditional cultures that ban the dead from the world of the living do so because of a belief that if the dead are not kept in their place, they will return to make trouble (Bendann 1930). The typical fear is that reminders of the dead will upset not the living but the dead. They are sad to have to leave the world of the living, wish to return and need to be told in no uncertain terms that they cannot. The dead are constructed as existing and needing to be kept in their place: overtures from the living will only encourage them to hang around. The leaving of food and drink by the grave, common in many cultures, ensures that the dead are well provided for in the next world, not least so that they will not come back to this world for sustenance and haunt the living. Some British folk beliefs about ghosts may well have a similar source (Finucane 1982), along with the desire to keep the dead in their place by placing a heavy tombstone on the grave. Those who died problematic deaths are in particular need of being kept away. The English custom of burying suicides at a cross-roads is intended to confuse the dead, who would not know the way home – comparable perhaps to the Shona custom in Zimbabwe of refusing the status of ancestor to villains and blackguards, ritually sending their spirit into a scapegoat and then driving the goat from the village and away into the bush.

Rosenblatt's 'reminder theory' explains these customs in terms of the psychological needs of the bereaved rather than the spiritual needs of the dead (Rosenblatt 1983: 39–40; Rosenblatt *et al.* 1976: ch.4). He argues that there is much to be said for banning, or at least limiting, reminders of the dead, whether by excluding them from conversation, getting rid of familiar artefacts or avoiding places they frequented while alive. Such reminders keep the memory of the dead alive and make it harder for the bereaved to move on to new relationships. In her study of American widows, Silverman (1986) found that grief was often harder and longer for the housewife widow who every minute is reminded of her husband as she moves around the house than it was for the working widow who, for some hours at least, could escape into the workplace. Likewise, with non-mortal kinds of loss: it can be harder for the dumped girl who sees her ex-boyfriend every day in class than for the one who never sees her ex again. In his study of nineteenth-century American diaries, Rosenblatt (1983) concluded that when a man left his woman to travel out West, it was often harder for her, daily surrounded by tangible reminders, than for him in a new world containing no reminders. Popular advice to bereaved people today to go out and get a job or find other distractions may be well founded.

There is also the possibility of a middle way, experienced by Silverman's working widows, of an oscillation between situations where the deceased seems ever present (the home) and situations where he is absent (work). With the typically modern separation of home and work (and, for the student, home and college), this oscillation between painful reminders and blessed escape is increasingly normal.[1] In smaller and more integrated tribal societies, separating bereaved people from reminders of the deceased may be more difficult to achieve and may require rituals such as the burning of the deceased's possessions or bans on mentioning the name of the dead. There will be enough reminders around anyway.

The trouble with this kind of explanation, however, is that although it ties in well with nineteenth- and twentieth-century popular wisdom about the need for distractions and with contemporary psychologies that recommend 'letting go', it does not relate to the subjective meanings given to avoidance in many non-western societies. These often concern the spiritual need of the dead to move on and the spiritual need of the living not to be haunted by the dead. Western psychology should not be applied to non-western experience without first taking into account indigenous interpretations of that experience, just as non-western mourning rituals cannot be transferred to the contemporary West without changing their meaning.

Rites of passage

Many traditional cultures, whether they encourage dialogues with the dead or whether they push the dead away, make clear that the dead are potentially dangerous and need handling with care. Those associated with the dead – the bereaved and those (Parry 1994) who handle the corpse – are, by association, also polluted. It may be no coincidence that they are, often, women (Bloch 1982: 226), femaleness being the gender often associated with pollution. The rituals that surround death, according to many anthropologists, deal with such matters of pollution and marginality.

Rites of passage have spawned a number of theories; here I will refer primarily to the most influential, developed by Arnold van Gennep in the first decade of the twentieth century but not translated into English until 1960. During the mourning period, both the bereaved and the deceased are, in Turner's (1977) phrase, betwixt and between. The dead are no longer alive, nor wholly passed over into the land of the dead; the bereaved are likewise caught between the world of the living and that of the dead. For van Gennep, funeral and mourning rituals move both the deceased and the bereaved into, through and beyond this marginal state. The rites transport the deceased to the land of the dead and the bereaved back to the land of the living. The bereaved, emotionally unbalanced, polluted by association with the dead, are kept out of play for a prescribed period, partly to protect the rest of the community from the taint of death, and partly to enable everyone concerned to adjust to new roles and identities. The middle – or liminal – phase of mourning, in which the bereaved are separated from society, is initiated by a rite of separation and ended by a rite of reincorporation back into society.

This links with Hertz's (1960) observation about double burial, which is the norm in the majority of cultures around the world. In cross-cultural terms the single burial performed in the contemporary English-speaking world is unusual. More typical is a wet funeral (the burial of the corpse), followed some years later by a dry funeral (the disinterment and relocation of the dry bones), as we have already seen is the case in rural Greece. In Hong Kong, at the final funeral the bones are placed in an earthenware pot, which is then buried – hence creating, to untutored western eyes, remarkably small grave plots in the cemeteries that adorn the hillsides. The two funerals demarcate the period in which the spirit of the dead, and the social existence of the bereaved, are 'betwixt and between'.[2]

Williams (1981) makes the important point that this three-stage model *describes* what often goes on in many traditional societies; van Gennep did not intend to *prescribe*. Yet this is precisely what many would-be reformers of the western way of grief have done. For them, western mourning is ineffective because it is not ritually marked into three stages: the brief once-only affair of the Anglo/American funeral is believed to leave the mourner adrift and alone with no further ritual markers. Although it seems logical that people need a period in which to adjust to change, there is little evidence that everyone does actually need a ritually defined mourning period. This may be because different individuals grieve in different ways and according to different timetables (Wortman and Silver 1989) and no imposed style of mourning can suit every individual. Indeed, there is historical evidence of people objecting to required ritual mourning, as with late Victorian women who saw it as limiting their personal freedom (see Chapter 7); many tripartite mourning rituals seem designed more to assist the dead and the power structure of society than the bereaved individual. But there are instances where the collapse of mourning rituals does seem to have left bereaved individuals at a loss, a good example being the early Jewish kibbutzim where the socialist kibbutz members rejected the religious symbolism of the Jewish funeral, with nothing to replace it (Rubin 1982, 1986).

There is also a tendency to see three-part rituals in the complex data from all traditional societies and cultures (including minority religious cultures in the modern West, such as Hinduism and Judaism), and never in mainstream contemporary white culture. In practice, the data is more complex. Following the Jewish funeral, the seven days of *shiva*, in which close relatives stay at home and are visited and brought food by more distant relatives, friends and neighbours, seems a perfect case of a liminal, out-of-play, period; yet it is followed by a further two periods of progressively reduced mourning, for 30 days, and then for a year, followed by yearly remembrances. This does not neatly fit van Gennep's model, for the Jewish rituals entail a number of liminal periods of varying lengths, nested within each other. Moreover, one may discern tripartite mourning structures in the modern West, even without formal ritual marking. Silverman's study of American widows (1986) observed a three-stage transition from wife to widow to woman, the intermediary identity of widow being one that many were unwilling to embrace. What encouraged them into and out of this identity was not religious ritual, but a mutual help group.

Social structure

So far in this chapter, I have been looking at some ways in which culture and religion affect relations between the living and the dead and how they are symbolized and ritualized in traditional societies. In this section, I look briefly at social and demographic structure, each of which can have a profound effect on relations with the dead.

Those critics of the modern way of death who like to think that 'natural is best' are inclined to believe that the nearer a society is to nature the more van Gennepian will be its death and mourning rituals. Not so. Immediate-return hunter-gatherer groups have minimal burial and mourning rituals (Woodburn 1982), more akin to minimalist modern British funerals than to the elaborate rituals documented by anthropologists in settled agricultural societies. The reason is simple. Funeral ritual has much to do with the distribution of property and power (Goody 1962). In hunter-gatherer societies, which depend on the ability to up and move camp to follow the rains, property is baggage that weighs you down, a liability rather than an asset; so property is minimal, and there is little to hand down on death. Because property is minimal and groups need to be small in order to be mobile, power differentials within society are also minimal, so one does not find grand aristocratic or royal funerals in which power has to be handed over, funerals which in agrarian societies have attracted the attention of anthropologists and historians. Another group – pastoralists – may, like hunter-gatherers, be nomads yet they own property (in the form of animals) and may have elaborate funerals; but the dead are left behind in their graves as the living continue their nomadic way. Such is the case with the gypsies (Okely 1983).

Something rather similar to hunter-gatherer mourning occurs in affluent modern societies. Most of those who die are elderly, have long since educated their offspring and have thereby passed on the knowledge that is the basis of power and prestige in modern society. The modern funeral of an old person therefore has little work to do. The family may read the will with interest, wondering who will inherit the house, but those fortunate enough to inherit are themselves already likely to be property owners and have been self-sufficient for some time.

Size of community can have a critical effect on mourning. In very small communities, the death of any one member affects everyone, while in a band numbering only a few dozen an accident, skirmish or epidemic that kills a dozen can be catastrophic. The group is weakened by death. Without bureaucratic systems that can easily replace any one worker, the unique skills of an individual may also be missed. People are also likely to die in harness, leaving a considerable gap. All this means that, though close kin may well grieve more than those distantly related to the deceased, the whole community mourns the loss. Known by all, the deceased can become an ancestor shared by all – if the belief system allows for this.

Blauner (1966) has pointed out how different the situation is in affluent, modern societies. People are (thankfully) likely to die in old age, having retired from work and reared their children, leaving no significant gap for economy and society to fill. Indeed, given the low status of the elderly in contemporary western society, their passing may hardly be noticed.[3] But their passing is most certainly noted by the remaining spouse, who after an intensely companionable marriage of 50 years, may be more attached to the deceased than are spouses in societies with much lower life expectancies and more diffuse kin relationships. The same may be true of today's children, who may likewise have known their parents for 50 years before death separates them. So in the modern situation, there is typically a huge gulf between a very few individuals who grieve long and deeply, and a penumbra of friends, neighbours and distant relatives who talk of comforting the bereaved, rather than of shared ancestors. This 'privatization' of grief is perhaps the most important historical development affecting bereavement today, and is a recurring theme in this book.

Only occasionally today does this privatization collapse, typically following a tragedy, disaster or high-profile death. If a school child dies, the whole school is shocked, including many children and teachers who did not know the child personally. In 1963 President Kennedy was assassinated and the entire American nation mourned. In 1986 the Challenger space shuttle, carrying teacher Christa McAuliffe along with the prospect of her giving lessons live from space to the nation's children, exploded on take-off, and millions grieved together – grieving perhaps as much the loss of a dream, a dream of American technological supremacy, safety through technique and the innocence of children. The communal mourning following the death of Princess Diana also displayed such characteristics. In these cases, communal loss by the group leads to large-scale funeral rituals, even in modern societies that have grown used to private mourning and slimline rituals. When an entire group is shattered by death, communal ritual and group mourning are brought out of the hat at a moment's notice.

This can lead to bemusement. Modern Britons are so used to the idea that you grieve only those you were personally close to, that following Princess Diana's death there was considerable perplexity at the scale of mourning for a princess most had never met. This was criticized as inauthentic, explicable only in terms of media manipulation. In fact, socially required mourning for one of high status, irrespective of personal connection, is more common in cultures around the world than is the Anglo/American notion of grieving only those to whom you are personally close. The response to Diana's death was certainly unusual for late twentieth-century Britons, but hardly inexplicable.

I do not mean to give the impression that small-scale societies always grieve communally. Much depends on culture, religion, power and status. The death of a pauper in Protestant early modern England, even though taking place in a small village, could be a miserable affair, attended by few. In such a case, marginal status plus a religion that had difficulty articulating relations between the living and the dead overcame the potential of small communities to mourn their own. The pauper had been a drain on the community and was not missed, and early Protestantism refused to assist the passage to heaven once a person has died. To become an ancestor, you need a religion and a culture that allows this as well as a group whose every member knew the deceased. This is why Princess Diana speedily became a publicly shared ancestor, and why the Puritan pauper did not and why the present writer – and most likely the present reader – will not.

If ancestors require small communities and an amenable religion, then we must ask in what sense and under what conditions is it possible to have ancestors in the modern West? The past few centuries have witnessed increasingly large connurbations in which individuals can know only a small proportion of the total population, an increasingly differentiated social structure, increasing individualism, and – in Western Europe at least – secularization. How can such a society relate to its dead? Before examining the evidence in Chapters 2–6, I first sketch some key developments in the West from the sixteenth to the nineteenth centuries that undermined medieval mourning and made the twentieth-century approach to bereavement possible.

Banishing the dead

For medieval people, life and especially religion were in large measure a matter – to borrow the title of Geary's book (1994) – of living with the dead. There was constant traffic between the two worlds, with the living praying to the saints on behalf of the newly dead so that they could be assisted through purgatory as painlessly and swiftly as possible, while the dead – in the person of the saints – could in turn assist the living. This process was increasingly controlled by the church, which used it to exercise power over the lives of individuals and communities. Prayers for the dead were offered in church, and if the dead were to speak it would be through priest or monk. As Roman Christianity spread north, the relics of saints associated with Rome were brought in to replace local saints, so the cult of the dead was used by Rome to increase its authority over the periphery.

The anti-papal nationalism behind the Protestant revolt meant that Rome's control of the dead needed to be broken. The existence of purgatory was denied; only heaven or hell were allowed as after-death possibilities. Indulgences (the trigger for the Reformation) were meaningless as were prayers, masses, alms for the dead and appeals to the saints. All medieval manifestations of communion between the living and the dead were swept away. The Reformation pronounced Jesus as the only intermediary between man and

God, at a stroke denying ordinary people intercourse between the living and the dead (Duffy 1992).

Early Protestant funerals might affirm the faith of the living, or challenge them to prepare themselves to meet their Maker, but in no way could they help the dead. This paved the way for the twentieth-century idea that funerals are not for the dead but for the living. The Anglican funeral service is, in fact, just the last few minutes of the lengthy Catholic requiem mass: the committal to the earth, without the mass. The Protestant funeral, *as funeral*, actually has no theology; it has no ritual efficacy in assisting the passage of the deceased to heaven, in the way that, for example, baptism in many Protestant churches inducts the believer into membership of the church. This vacuum left the Protestant funeral wide open to co-option by new meanings and new interest groups.

Secular feasting took the place of extensive religious ritual. This was reflected in a shift in costs from paying for the priest to paying for food and alcohol:

The funeral of George Glandish, of Ebony Court, Kent, in 1622, cost a total of £6 6s 5d. Of this sum, £5 1s 9d was spent on a feast at Ebony Court after the interment, for which the following items were bought: 2 sides of mutton, 6 bushels of wheat, 6 pounds of currants, half a pound of sugar, 1 ounce of cloves and mace, 1 ounce of cinnamon, butter, a fat calf, 12 pounds of bacon, 40 pounds of cheese, a fat wether, 7 dozen and 2 loaves, 23 twopenny loaves and beer. The remaining £1 4s 8d was ample to provide a simple coffin and shroud and to pay the fees of the minister, clerk, sexton, bearers and bell-ringers, as well as any other incidental expenses.

(Gittings 1984: 97)

The funeral became more an opportunity to display earthly status than heavenly destination.

Starting at the end of the seventeenth century, and gathering pace in the nineteenth, the new undertaking profession shifted the marks of status away from food and drink toward the funeral procession itself. By 1800, one London burial club allocated no money for food, but contracted with the undertaker to supply:

a strong elm coffin covered with superfine black and furnished with two rows all round, close drove, with best black japanned nails and adorned with rich ornamental drops, a handsome plate of inscription, angel above the plate, flower beneath, and four pair of handsome handles, with wrought grips; the coffin to be well-pitched, lined and ruffled with crepe, a handsome crape shroud, cap and pillow. For use, a handsome velvet pall, three gentlemen's cloaks, three crape hatbands, three hoods and scarves, and six pairs of gloves, two porters equipped to attend the funeral, a man to attend the same with hat and gloves; also the burial fees paid if not exceeding one guinea.

(quoted in Gittings 1984: 97)

By the mid-nineteenth century, public health as much as status governed burial. The well-worn medieval pattern of burial, suitable for village church-yards with relatively static populations, broke down under the pressure of population growth and the high death rate that characterized the new in-dustrial towns and thriving capital cities (notably Paris and London). Burial came to be perceived as public health hazard number one, and new rational systems for burial – bolstered by a whole raft of new legislation – came into force (Curl 1980). The development of cremation in the twentieth century was likewise seen, at least to some extent, as a public health measure.

By the beginning of the twentieth century, western (especially Protestant) funeral practice was determined not by the spiritual needs of the dead but by status and public health. The twentieth century added to these the com-fort of the bereaved, first through religious liturgies that played down sin and worms and played up the comforting twenty-third psalm (Farrell 1980: ch.5), and later through the idea that the funeral is an important part of the grief process, an idea particularly fashionable in the USA (and mercilessly pilloried in 1963 by Jessica Mitford's *The American Way of Death*). Over four centuries, the dead have effectively been removed from the Protestant funeral, though they are still there in Catholic and Orthodox funerals. For Protestants, and even more for those with no religious faith at all, what matters is not to assist the dead in the passage to heaven, but the gastro-nomy, status, physical health, spiritual comfort and psychological health of the living. Geary (1994: 1–2) observes 'The dead are banished ... never before have humans been able to kill so many people so efficiently or to forget them so completely.'

The celebration of grief

I have already mentioned that as social groupings become bigger, not every member will have known the deceased or have been affected by his or her death, so that a distinction arises between 'the bereaved' and everyone else. Bereavement becomes a psychological experience of the individual, rather than the shared experience of the group; individual grief replaces group mourning. This is particularly so when the nuclear family rather than the wider kin group is the main point of reference. Romantic love has been documented for at least 2500 years (Mount 1982) and the nuclear family has been the norm in England way back into the Middle Ages, but the Victorian period positively celebrated marital affection and encouraged individuals – especially women – to invest all their emotional energies in spouse and children. The romantic movement added to this the injunction

to marry for love not money, an injunction that became ever more pronounced in the twentieth century. The end of millennium popularity of film
versions of nineteenth-century English romantic novels testifies both to the
continuing celebration of romantic love and to its historical source.

French historian Philippe Ariès argues, and I agree with him, that this
led in the nineteenth century to an obsession with the death of the other.
If the late medieval and early modern preoccupation was 'what will happen
to me and my loved ones when we die?', the nineteenth- (and twentieth-)
century concern has primarily been 'how will I cope when my beloved
dies?' The answer was through a grief that reflected and demonstrated the
eternal bond with the deceased, and a faith in an ultimate reunion in heaven.
In this sense, bereavement is an invention of the romantic movement:

> Beginning in the eighteenth century, affectivity was, from childhood,
> entirely concentrated on a few individuals, who became exceptional,
> irreplaceable, and inseparable. 'One person is absent, and the whole
> world is empty' . . . Today there is a tendency to regard romanticism as
> an aesthetic and bourgeois mode, without depth. We now know that it
> is a major objective fact of daily life, a profound transformation of
> man as a social being.
>
> (Ariès 1981: 472)

I would not say that people did not grieve before this period – that mani-
festly is not so – but what became new was grief's celebration, first in
Victorian sentimentality and now, a century later, in self-help bereavement
literature.

If they were to celebrate, to indulge in, grief, Victorians required leisure.
The working-class widow could not afford a lengthy period of mourning:
she needed to continue to work, to bring up her children and find a replacement husband as soon as possible. It was the upper and upper middle-
classes, and in particular the women of these classes, who had the leisure
to obey the new mourning rules and absent themselves from social life for a
period of months. With servants and husbands to labour for them, they
were in any case already excused from the day-to-day responsibilities of
childcare and earning a living (Morley 1971; Jalland, in press). Some Victorians used their leisure time to contact the dear departed through spiritualist
mediums, who originate from this period (Moore 1975; Barrow 1986; Owen
1989).

As well as leisure, indulging in grief also requires privacy. This has been
highlighted by Lofland, commenting on the twentieth century, but one can
see the origins of the phenomenon in the nineteenth:

> The modern literature on grief is replete with descriptions of private
> activities in which bereaved persons engage which keep their attention
> riveted to their loss. Quite typically and literally, they seek the lost

person. Taking long solitary walks, scanning faces for a glimpse of the dead other is not unusual behaviour . . . They visit places and look at objects rich in association with the lost other; going over photographs again and again, or returning repeatedly to a particular cafe . . . These behaviour patterns among the bereaved . . . could only occur among persons who have access to considerable periods of solitude and privacy and who have considerable time and space discretion.

(Lofland 1985: 180)

Such grieving cannot take place in a single-room dwelling with five or ten occupants – the typical living arrangement of the poor in the nineteenth and previous centuries. Immersion in grief is a luxury only to be afforded by those with the requisite time and space.

The Victorian celebration of female grief, together with leisure and privacy, meant that upper- and some middle-class ladies were able to live in companionship with the dead for an entire year of mourning or, in the case of Queen Victoria, for 40 (Stroebe *et al.* 1992). Whereas Stroebe and Schut (1999) argue that mourning entails an oscillation between immersion in the emotional work of grief and having to engage in practical tasks, the serious-minded Victorian widow could abandon practical life and indulge her sorrow. Furthermore she would be respected for it, as George Eliot satirized in *The Mill on the Floss*:

It was not everybody who could afford to cry so much about their neighbours who had left them nothing; but Mrs Pullet had married a gentleman farmer, and had leisure and money to carry her crying and everything else to the highest degree of respectability.

Meanwhile upper-class Victorian males were expected to distract themselves by throwing themselves into their work (Jalland 1996: 4–5). Which is not to say that men did not grieve. Widower William Barnes, for one, lived in the romantic world of the dead:

In every moaning wind I hear thee say
sweet words of consolation . . .
I live, I talk with thee wheree'er I stray

(in Stallworthy 1973: 361–2)

Such mourners felt it was a betrayal of their love to think that grief would ever end. Romanticism demanded a relationship with the beloved beyond the grave (Rosenblatt 1983; Stroebe *et al.* 1992).

By the end of the century, however, upper-class ladies were beginning to reject the world of the dead into which they were cast. Mourning periods steadily reduced, upper- and upper middle-class ladies wished to think for themselves and be free to grieve as felt right to them as individuals rather than as socially prescribed, and there was a gathering reaction against what was increasingly seen as the morbidness of living with the dead (Cannadine 1981; Taylor 1983). The First World War dealt the final blow to Victorian mourning, as there was no way that women of any class could spend the rest of the war in mourning: they had to work in the munitions factories and in the fields, and staff the field hospitals. If the nineteenth century (for the well-to-do at least) was characterized by romantic association with the recent dead, the twentieth century quickly came to see all this as morbid, embracing instead the everyday attitude of the here-and-now, though spiritualism continued to flourish till mid century.

Yet all consuming grief would not go away. Passionate grief was to blossom again in the second half of the twentieth century, not in the guise of romantic communion with the dead but in the guise of a modernist psychology of grief that inherited from Victorian romanticism a preoccupation with the emotions but that left behind the dead themselves (see Chapter 6).

Summary

This chapter has sketched relations between the living and the dead in more traditional societies, including previous centuries in the West. First, the dialogues with the ancestors that are conducted in many traditional societies are introduced, along with the religious language in which these dialogues are typically conducted. In other traditional societies, however, conversing with the dead is not allowed – whether to minimize reminders to the dead of the world they have left, or to minimize reminders to the living of the ones they have lost. The marginal status of the bereaved, betwixt and between the living and the dead, then leads to a brief discussion of Hertz, van Gennep and Turner's theories concerning rites of passage. Though the permission of religion and culture is necessary if ancestors are to be created, another pre-requisite is a settled and small-scale society in which the dead are well known to the entire group. Without this, group mourning typically becomes the private grief so familiar in the modern West, a transition further facilitated by the Reformation's ban on communing with the dead. Victorian Romanticism, however, celebrated the eternal bond with the dead, even if this bond was entirely private to the one left behind.

Further reading

Ariès, P. (1974) *Western Attitudes toward Death: From the Middle Ages to the Present*. Baltimore: Johns Hopkins University Press. (London: Marion Boyars, 1994)

Danforth, L. (1982) *The Death Rituals of Rural Greece*. Princeton, NJ: Princeton University Press.
Geary, P.J. (1994) *Living with the Dead in the Middle Ages*. Ithaca: Cornell University Press.
Huntington, R. and Metcalf, P. (1992) *Celebrations of Death: The Anthropology of Mortuary Ritual*, 2nd edn. Cambridge: Cambridge University Press.
Morley, J. (1971) *Death, Heaven and the Victorians*. London: Studio Vista.

Questions

1 Who do you know from non-western cultures? Ask them whether bonds with the dead should be broken, or maintained.
2 Do funeral and mourning rituals in your own society have a three-part structure?

Notes

1 This is related to, but not exactly the same as, the oscillation to which Stroebe and Schut (1999) refer.
2 Though in rural Greece (Danforth 1982) and in Naples (Pardo 1989) the second burial is ritually marked, in much of Europe this is not the case and it does not mark the end of mourning; it is simply a practicality required by the need to re-use the grave for a new occupant (Goody and Poppi 1994).
3 Disengagement theory (Cumming and Henry 1961) argues, somewhat controversially, that the marginalization of the elderly is *due* to the fact that they are likely to die. Reducing their importance to society reduces the consequences of their eventual demise. A corollary is that in societies with high death rates, where death is typically of the young, it is the young that are seen as unimportant.

2 War, peace and the dead: twentieth-century popular culture

Better by far you should forget and smile
Than that you should remember and be sad
(Christina Rossetti)

At the going down of the sun and in the morning we will remember them.
(Lawrence Binyon)

The history of bereavement in the twentieth century has yet to be written. A few historians have researched loss through war (Winter 1995; Bourke 1996), but Cannadine (1981), Merridale (forthcoming) and psychoanalysts Alexander and Margarete Mitscherlich (1975) are unusual in examining the impact of wartime loss on subsequent peacetime culture – looking at Britain, the Soviet Union and Germany respectively. In this chapter, I will sketch how popular thinking about the desirability of continuing versus breaking bonds with the dead seems to have evolved during the twentieth century.

WAR

Winter (1997) has argued that there are three forms of memory utilized by those who have survived battle: forgetting, remembering and what was once called shell shock but what, since Vietnam, has come to be known as post-traumatic stress disorder (PTSD) (Healy 1993; Young 1995). In PTSD, intrusive images and thoughts and the compulsion to replay old events force the past into the present; in defence, sufferers protect themselves by avoiding any triggers to memory, for instance through substance abuse. In PTSD, forgetting and remembering interact painfully and chaotically, and incapacitate the sufferer. Although grief and dealing with traumatic memo-ries are not the same thing, Winter's three categories of forgetting, remember-ing and incapacitating distress may be loosely used to suggest three ways of dealing with the stress and grief that twentieth-century war has prompted.

Forgetting

In 1915, a British corporal in a convalescent home wrote this in an auto-graph book:

> I have been asked to write an account of my experiences in France and Belgium. To tell the truth, I would rather not, as they to me are best forgotten. I can only describe modern warfare as horrible in the extreme and I'm sure all will agree, that such incidents as are daily witnessed in the line should be forgotten as quickly as possible.
>
> (Bourke 1996: 22)

Forgetting is perhaps the most common response of the fighting man and of bombed and occupied civilians. When called upon to fight, or to provide moral support for those doing the fighting, they *have* to forget: wallowing in grief will undermine fighting performance. (Much the same is true of doctors and nurses in emergency wards.) Even when there is more leisure, as for the corporal in the convalescent home or after the war, many *choose* to forget. Not just in letters home from the front, but on leave and after demobilization the soldier may choose to tell his wife little or nothing of the deepest experiences of his life. She in turn may choose not to tell him about the privations at home or of her worries, since the wartime ethic is to keep cheerful and encourage those away fighting. Adjusting to peacetime means leaving the past behind. In continental Europe, silence might in addi-tion cover situations such as unwanted sexual advances from occupying troops or near starvation. This sets up a pattern in families in which stress, by women as well as by men, is coped with by not talking about it. Society as well as individuals and families can also choose to forget. Popular and official images, especially after 1945 in Britain, depicted a clean war 'where people died intact and quickly; where the injured overcame their disabil-ities; where cheerful, patriotic wives and sweethearts waited patiently and faithfully back home' (Bender 1997: 343). This too covered up the truth.

Children in the inter-war period typically had parents who chose to re-main silent about wartime experience and who bore the depression of the 1930s with quiet stoicism; these children were then required to fight in the Second World War, confirming the necessity for courageous silence. They brought up their own children, my generation, with little reference to the past and with few stories of deceased family members, least of all stories of those who died traumatically. Now elderly, they (like more recent survivors of disaster) may find unwanted reminders (such as war movies or high profile fiftieth anniversary commemorations of D-Day or of the end of the war) painful, especially when these reminders sanitize the war and distort the person's own life history (Bender 1997). They may also be bemused by what they see as end-of-century fads for family history and for expressing grief.

Bender (1997) argues that they may also be bemused by the current fashion in gerontology for reminiscence work. Since the 1980s, group reminiscence has become popular in old people's homes, the aim originally being to stimulate deteriorating memory but, in the hands of poorly trained staff, reminiscence sessions have degenerated into mere entertainment. How do old people in reminiscence groups in residential homes respond to this?

> In practice, members often take one look at the untrained staff who have had no teaching about group work; assess their age, experience and style; and decide that the best they can get out of the group is a round of 'Good Old Days' and 'Poor but happy'. Intellectually and emotionally, all that is on offer is akin to junk food.
>
> (Bender 1997: 345)

Even the experts who write on reminiscence, such as Erikson *et al.* (1986), often ignore the painful memories that old people may not wish to dredge up.

There is evidence that those Holocaust survivors who have subsequently coped best with life have been those who did not talk about their experiences. In one study of survivors' coping mechanisms,

> The well-adjusted survivors displayed a repressive tendency in their daily life-style. Most of them had not talked all these years about the Holocaust. In some cases, the avoidance was so dominant that even their close relatives barely knew anything about their experiences during that period, if they even knew at all that the survivors had actually lived through the Holocaust. By their own testimony, this does not mean they have forgotten what happened to them during the Holocaust; they have just avoided, both in wakefulness and in sleep, the recurrent penetration of the feelings that they had felt during their confinement.
>
> (Kaminer and Lavie 1993: 345)

The Mitscherlichs (1975) argue that post-war Germans have coped by an almost wholesale forgetting of their enthusiasm for Hitler and even of the scale of their defeat. Colin Murray Parkes has observed that it is not just in the contemporary West that war may be coped with by forgetting.[1] His impressions are that throughout the world, warlike people choose not to speak of the dead. The silence of the Apaches about their dead, mentioned in Chapter 1, may be due to a history of war. In Rwanda, Parkes attended a mass funeral where the only person who showed any emotion was not from that country, torn by genocide, but from relatively peaceful East Africa. Cross-cultural research is needed, however, to test Parkes's hypothesis.

If he is right, then we may postulate the following: (1) Victorian communion with the dead required not only leisure and privacy, but also the 99 years of relative peace that reigned from 1815 to 1914; (2) the twentieth-century European reserve about speaking of grief arose, at least in part, from two specific generations that fought in the two World Wars; (3) only now in the second half of the twentieth century, with two generations that have not personally experienced war, are people in countries such as the UK likely to be more open about grief and to be more willing to speak of those who have died; and (4) there may be important differences in grieving styles between currently middle aged Americans (and Australians) who fought in Vietnam and those (often more educated) who avoided the draft.

Remembrance and remembering

Those fighting a war who suffer multiple bereavements may grieve surprisingly little and may do their best to forget. But here's a paradox, for western societies at large remember their war dead better than their civilians. It is only the war dead whose names are inscribed for all to see on prominent memorials, whether an English village war memorial, the Vietnam Veterans Memorial in Washington DC, or the national war memorial in Canberra. No one dies on active service without their name being carved in stone for posterity. (By contrast, unless they die in the course of a civil war, civilians are typically not memorialized publicly.) The Commonwealth War Graves Commission has comprehensive records of the graves and memorials for all Commonwealth service personnel who have died on active service since 1914, enabling relatives to find the site and visit. Only those who die in war can thus be found. Moreover, every year, the war dead are collectively remembered, whether in the British Remembrance Sunday or the American Memorial Day (Warner 1959: ch.8). Indeed, since 1995, the ritual remembrance of the British war dead has actually been expanded, with many supermarkets, work places and colleges now marking a two-minute silence not only on Remembrance Sunday but also on November 11th. Civilians do not find the entire nation stopping to remember them, decades after their death.[2] But in civil wars around the world, from the USA to Northern Ireland to El Salvador, the civilian as well as the military dead may live on as patriotic and/or anti-regime symbols for years, or even centuries, later (Kearl and Rinaldi 1983; Schwartz 1990).

Memorials and rituals for the war dead not only remember them, but also define the group, whether it be the Vietnam generation, Australian national identity, or the local English village. The London suburb of North-wood where I grew up, green fields until the late nineteenth century when a straggle of shops and houses began to spread out from the Metropolitan Railway station, had no symbolic focus until the First World War memorial was built; it was the death of its young men that turned this pleasantly convenient dormitory into a community with a history and a (broken) heart. To this day, the memorial remains as the only symbol of Northwood, the one place where people might instinctively gather at times of crisis. Other places where people gather are merely functional, economically or socially: the station, the shops, the pubs, even the various churches.

Winter (1997), however, argues that though nations can engage in ritual acts of remembrance, they cannot remember. As a child in the 1950s attending Remembrance Day ceremonies at the war memorial, I was engaging in an act of remembrance, but I did not remember. Only individuals, families and small groups who share a common experience can remember.

This is movingly expressed in Vera Brittain's autobiography *Testament of Youth* (1933) about her experiences in the First World War. She corresponds with her fiancé Roland, who is fighting abroad; in one letter, she is furious with him for seeming to forget her and for being absorbed with life in the trenches. He is killed, the day before being due home on leave. Later, she goes to work as a nurse at a field dressing station in northern France and for the first time begins to understand: she resents having to go home to care for her ailing mother, a trifling task compared with the real work to be done in France. Her bonds with the sick and the dying in France are now stronger than those with her own family. In the final chapter, she describes her eventual post-war courtship with another man, her disillusion with the inferior males that the war left alive, the inability of those only three or four years younger to comprehend, and her reluctance to marry, lest it break faith with Roland. Yet she rises to the challenge of facing the future and starting again, without forgetting the past.

Thus the war produced what Winter terms fictive kinship groups and what Seale (1998), following Anderson (1991), terms imagined communities. Groups which go through terrible times together can choose to construct a collective memory that is denied their biological and legal kin. Members of veterans' associations may drink together every week. They may share memories, or they may collectively find memories too awful to talk about, but either way they are in the company of men who know what it was like. Symbolizing the fictive kinship group is the British tradition of service personnel being buried where they fell, with their comrades, rather than in a family plot back home. Ex-servicemen's pilgrimages to the old battlefields and their associated cemeteries boomed in the 1980s and 1990s (Walter 1993c). But if the fictive kinship group ceases to meet, if its members cease to lower the flag or blow the bugle at sunset, to drink together, to go on pilgrimage together, their collective memory will fade.

I return to fictive kinship groups in Chapter 11 where I discuss mutual help bereavement groups. But just as peacetime memory of the dead need not be within such a group, nor need wartime memory. Many remembered in private ways. Thousands of widows, fiancées and mothers, as well as veterans, visited overseas war cemeteries in the 1920s, sometimes on their own, often on organized tours. Cannadine (1981) has described how spiritualist mediums were regularly consulted throughout the inter-war period. Spiritualism's most effective convert was the novelist, Sir Arthur Conan Doyle, who joined the movement in 1916 after losing a son in the war. Spiritualism declined in popularity only from the 1950s, but to this day a number of bereaved parents consult a medium in order to be reassured that their child is at peace.

The inability to mourn

Whether the response was to forget or to remember, Cannadine (1981) and Winter (1995) disagree with those such as Gorer (1965) and Ariès (1981) who claim that the First World War precipitated a twentieth-century denial of death. There was remembering as well as forgetting, speaking as well as refusing to speak. Winter argues that well-worn Victorian motifs were able to articulate the unimaginable losses suffered, not least among these being spiritualism, the identification of the dead soldier with the crucified Christ and the rather traditional design of war memorials.[3] The First World War was one in which the sufferings of both sides could be marked. For Winter, it was the Second World War that created unprecedented problems of memory. How could the dead of the Holocaust, of Hiroshima and Nagasaki be remembered? There is a literature of poetry and countless letters emerging from the gangrene and the rotting corpses of the First World War trenches, but where is the equivalent literature from Hiroshima and Nagasaki? How can a Jew remember, when there is no other member of his family left with whom to remember? How could the Soviet Union mourn the – it is now estimated – 60 million of its citizens who died from violence and hunger between 1917 and 1989, more than half of them in the wars of 1939–1945 (Merridale, forthcoming)?

If it is hard remembering the victims who died in such circumstances, it is impossible to remember those who killed them. Whereas in the First World War, soldiers might write to bereaved women on the opposing side, telling how their loved ones died, what memories could be respectfully shared by the Nazi or Japanese soldier, the concentration camp guard, the informer and the secret policeman? These are now the disgraced dead, men whom we neither remember nor choose to forget, but men whom we have to forget, creating what the Mitscherlichs (1975) describe as Germany's inability, following 1945, to mourn the Führer they had loved and followed.

Germany experienced a numbness, a failure to do the 'labour of grieving' and own up to the crimes of the Third Reich and lament all that it had destroyed.

Bergen, however, argues that post-war Germany was able to mourn, by turning its attention away from the men who fought and toward the women who suffered, away from the perpetrators of violence and toward its victims.

> By emphasizing the 'feminine past' – a wartime story of bombed-out homes, widowhood, and rape – Germans could mourn their own suffering even while they erased memories of the 'masculine' past – armed aggression, murderous bureaucracy, and genocidal slaughter – that had wrought massive destruction on others. In this way, comforting phrases and rituals of public mourning could coexist with silence and denial.
>
> (Bergen 1997)

If the Allies tended to be silent about the sufferings of its civilians, Germany's enforced silence about the sacrifices made by its soldiers may have enabled it to mourn and remember her civilian sufferings.

Remembering those Americans who died in Vietnam presents a not totally dissimilar problem, though on a far smaller scale. How can they be remembered when the cause they fought for has been subsequently discredited? After years of debate, the Vietnam Veterans Memorial was eventually built, to widespread though by no means universal acclaim, serving to honour the dead without necessarily honouring the war (Palmer 1988; Sellars and Walter 1993). Unlike so many war memorials that rise in defiant triumph high above the ground, the Vietnam memorial is sunk into the ground. As you walk down below the grass of the Mall, you pass the names of the 57,692 Americans who died, each carved into a low 492-foot wall of black marble, while in the polished stone you see the pale reflections of mourners. At places at the foot of the wall are flowers and messages and potted plants. One or two people lean over the top, pressing crayon on paper to get a tracing of the name they have been looking for. Unlike many memorials from earlier wars, where names are listed alphabetically within each battalion, at Washington the names are simply in chronological order of death. There is no regimental pride here, just 57,692 sets of individual pain. Seekers after a name are told which section theirs is in, and then they have to seek among the dead to find their man.

Vietnam is significant for a further reason, namely the identification in the late 1970s of post-traumatic stress disorder to account for the self-destructive and anti-social responses of many veterans to their war experiences (Young 1995). How could veterans mourn their part in atrocities that officially did not happen? Identifying PTSD was highly political, for it helped publicize atrocities committed by American troops and rendered the federal government responsible for mental as well as for physical disabilities deriving from battle. It also helped popularize the ideas that repressed trauma

LIBRARY, UNIVERSITY OF CHESTER

can cause subsequent pathology and that exploring the past in therapy can help people face the future.

One reason there may be an inability to mourn, to be discussed further in Chapter 5, is that knowledge of where and how a person died may be deliberately kept from relatives. This is most likely to occur in civil war. As I write, concerted efforts – from Chile, to Ireland, to South Africa – are being made to get this information. Only last month, following the recent Northern Ireland peace agreement, I read:

> IRA READY TO IDENTIFY GRAVES   The IRA is believed to be on the point of identifying the graves of about a dozen people it abducted and killed. The terrorist victims all disappeared between 1972 and 1980, but the many appeals from their families for the location of their bodies to be pinpointed have been rejected. Reports in Dublin, though, said the IRA leadership was ready to permit the remains to be returned. Gerry Adams, the Sinn Fein president, called on anyone with information about the 'disappeared' to come forward to help those families to put the tragedy behind them.
>
> (*The Times* 27 June 1998)

Systematic efforts of this kind at present are being made by South Africa's Truth and Reconciliation Commission (TRC), chaired by Desmond Tutu. The TRC believes that Nuremberg-style trials, in which prosecutions are aimed for, will prompt killers to avoid revealing the truth. The TRC believes, correctly or incorrectly, that most South Africans are more concerned to know what happened to their relatives than to exact retribution, so the TRC's method is to offer amnesty to those who agree to testify by a particular date. The Commission believes this is important for individuals who are grieving, and that it is important for the entire country – neither can come to terms with their present if they have not come to terms with their past. By this means, South Africa's history is literally being re-written, and the links between war, bereavement and the writing of history become manifest. Whether this will create a precedent for conflicts in other countries in future, only time will tell.

Whether the Holocaust, the Nazi period, Vietnam and civil wars throughout the world have created an 'inability to mourn' in certain generations in certain countries remains on open question. It indicates the danger of generalizing about the consequences of twentieth-century war for twentieth-century bereavement – each nation, each generation, each gender has its own experiences and ways of coping with them.

PEACE

Apart from war, a number of trends have affected the extent to which popular culture since 1945 has encouraged us to live with the dead or, more often, to leave them behind. Several of these trends began long before in earlier centuries.

Religion

One such concerns religious changes. The Victorian tendency to see heaven in terms of reunion with kin is still popular at the end of the twentieth century, and provides one of the major languages in which people, especially old people, speak of death and their relationships with those who have 'gone before' (McDannell and Lang 1988; Littlewood 1992: 109–14). Many elderly bereaved people have no intention of 'getting over it', looking forward instead to joining their dead husband or wife shortly. This may be hard for their middle aged children, who would rather mum went out and made a life for herself, but the 85-year-old's approach to her loss may be as rational as any, given physical weariness and a life expectancy, statistically, of no more than two or three more years.

Hope of reunion with kin has undermined the power of the churches. The more the afterlife is seen in terms of automatic reunion, the less people are willing to entertain the possibility that their dear beloved may not arrive at the right place. The concept of hell has been under philosophical and theological attack since the late seventeenth century (Walker 1964; Almond 1994), but at the popular level it was hell's incompatibility with automatic family reunion that led to its demise. The First World War, hell on earth, undermined eternal hell still further, it being impossible for padres even to hint that any of the brave young men they were burying on the field of battle had gone to the wrong place (Wilkinson 1978). From the 1920s onwards, most churches, including in the 1960s the Catholic church, downplayed sin and hell, not least in their funeral liturgies. After the 1960s, even conservative evangelicals such as Billy Graham were keeping quiet about hell, implying that non-believers did not go there but simply ceased to exist (Walter 1996a). With death no longer posing any great spiritual risk, death and the life after find less and less mention in sermons and church teaching. If Protestantism is historically premised on banning intercourse between this world and the next, by the end of the twentieth century it had virtually ceased to make any reference to the next world at all.

The churches' silence about the next life has, however, left a vacuum readily filled by conjectures (Walter 1993a). Belief in ghosts is the only religious belief held by more young Britons than by old Britons. Judging by the current wave of books and movies, angels, especially guardian angels, are also increasingly popular. The idea of the angelic dead looking after us may now be more popular than the old idea of the ghostly dead who make trouble. Contemporary angels are so new that social surveys have not yet added them to their list of questions about religious belief, so we do not

know for certain whether or not angels have yet ousted ghosts in the popularity stakes. The late twentieth century is a time when not only religion but
also science is looked at with some scepticism, opening the way for all
kinds of ideas to be entertained – from reincarnation to crop circles to
aliens to near death experiences. The brakes that first Protestantism and
then science imposed upon communing with the dead are now well and
truly released, and who knows what kind of post-mortem communions will
become possible in the third millennium?

Burial and cremation

The development of cremation in the West is related to religious trends.
Secular but historically Protestant countries such as Sweden and Britain
have high rates of cremation, contrasting markedly with religious Ulster,
and even more with religious *and* Catholic Eire. (Among western societies
with a low cremation rate, the only two that are not overwhelmingly Catholic
are Finland and the USA). Cremation has implications for communing with
the dead, for one of the major activities conducted by those who visit
graves is to talk to the deceased and generally to look after the dead by
keeping the grave in good order. This regularly happens in Britain, and
even without communal rituals of the kind we encountered in rural Greece
in the previous chapter, the Hertzian dynamic of relating to the deceased's
soul by caring for the resting place of his body still applies. Many still can
echo the sentiments of Emily Dickinson:

> The grave my little cottage is,
> where 'Keeping house' for thee
> I make my parlour orderly
> And lay the marble tea
> (Johnson 1970: 706, cited in Stroebe *et al.* 1992: 1208)

Well worn images are of the dead as sleeping and of the grave as a bed.
Kerbstones were particularly popular in the inter-war period, which together
with the headstone created an effect redolent of a bed. When the second
spouse is laid side by side, the double bed says it all about post-mortem
reunion.

With cremation, though, there is no grave to visit. This is not to say that
those who have been cremated cannot be spoken to, cared for and in many
other ways continue to play a part in the lives of the living – 86 per cent of
a representative sample of those living in the English county of Notting-
hamshire said that they did not think there was any difference between
burial and cremation as far as their memory of the dead was concerned
(Davies 1997: 158). But to go back to Hertz, without religious belief,

without a corpse lying in a grave, is it harder for the mourner to envisage relating to the dead? Does cremation make communion with the dead harder? Or have secular Protestant countries embraced cremation because they do not envisage communing with the dead, so may as well send the deceased up the crematorium chimney and be done with it? There may be something in both these possibilities (Jupp 1997).

What about the United States of America and Finland, the two oddities in the cremation league table? Here I would argue that burial remains popular because large numbers of their citizens desire links not only with the individual dead but also with all the family ancestors who represent their ethnic identity (Davies 1997: 100). Burial is particularly popular in the USA with the first few generations. This may in part be due to recent immigrants' religion (they are, for example, more likely to be Catholic), but burial also contains important symbolism. The graves of the family ancestors, grouped together with others of the same ethnic group in a special section of the cemetery, make a clear statement about the family's ethnic identity. But their location within a multi-cultural cemetery also symbolizes their membership of a multi-cultural America (Matturi 1993); below ground, the ancestors' symbolic preservation (through embalming, stout caskets and concrete grave liners) within the American soil like-wise indicates their enduring commitment to their new land (Walter 1993b). Any family member visiting the cemetery is clearly linked not only to the individual being visited, but to an entire family ancestry and its history.

Finland, not a country of immigrants, nevertheless also needs to keep touch with its past, more a matter for them of national than of ethnic identity. Independent only from 1917, with its two ex-colonizers (Sweden and Russia) on either side, this young country lost a disproportionate number in the Second World War. The graves of the war dead lying in the Finnish forest came to represent Finland itself, which then extended to a cult of the civilian dead too. Finland is still too precarious a country to let its dead go up the chimney to be blown who knows where. (Cremation is typically chosen for those whose family graves are full, the ashes being buried in the grave; burial would have been their first choice.) Both the USA and Finland exemplify Childe's thesis (1945) that it is those whose status is insecure who are likely to take most care over mortuary ritual and over memorializing their dead.

Social death

One way to understand the continuing bond with the dead is to say that, though physically dead, socially they may still be very much alive. Social and physical death, like social and physical birth, need not occur simultaneously (Mulkay 1993). In societies in which the ancestors play a significant role, social death may not occur until there is no one left alive who remembers the deceased, that is, another couple of generations or so. In contemporary western societies, the opposite is often the case: the confused geriatric patient may well have died socially long before dying physically. When this occurs, grief may also be played out long before death – the grief of middle aged children who have lost the mother they knew, even though her body lingers on interminably in the geriatric nursing home. This is often mistakenly called 'anticipatory grief', grief in anticipation of the loss of the person, but the truth is that the person is already lost: the family are grieving very much for a loss that has already occurred.

Dying socially before they die physically is the death that westerners fear most. At the same time, there are few publicly available languages that speak of social life after physical death, so the good death is now where social and physical death coincide. Promoting this kind of death is the mission of two movements that are otherwise at daggers drawn: the euthanasia and hospice (palliative care) movements. For the advocate of euthanasia, it is intolerable that someone should be kept physically alive if their personality has been destroyed through accident or disease such as Alzheimer's and/or they are in chronic, untreatable pain. They are psychologically and socially dead – why keep them alive physically? Euthanasia brings physical death forward in time, so that it can more nearly coincide with social death.

The palliative care movement, while promoting the same end (the coincidence of physical and social death), advocates the opposite means. It's motto is 'giving life to years, not years to life', by which is meant the treatment of pain (personal and spiritual as well as physical) so that the person can live as fully as possible until the day that physical death naturally arrives. Thus, palliative care extends social life so that the person remains socially alive as far as possible until the moment of physical death. Social life is extended not just for the patient as an individual, but by creating a setting – whether in hospice, home or hospital – in which staff, relatives and friends can relate to the person as a full, though physically dying, human being. In other words, it is a challenge to the institutionalization (Goffman 1968) that so often compounds the loss of social life wrought by some of the diseases of old age.

Some palliative care units memorialize the dead via memory books, candles and memorial services, and many provide bereavement services. In such ways, they encourage the social existence of the dead person to be maintained beyond the grave. The primary goal of palliative care, though, and the standard by which it asks to be judged, is the that of extending social life until the moment of physical death, rather than that of extending it beyond the grave.

Forgetting versus remembering

Romanticism, celebrating the continuing spirit of the deceased beloved, though out of fashion intellectually is still carried by popular culture. Though clergy and other burial authorities in Britain often discourage what they see as sentimental epitaphs, especially when familiar names (such as 'Dad') are proposed, some families succeed in inscribing their loved one's stone with sentiments such as:

> Those you love don't go away
> They walk beside you every day
> (Kensal Green cemetery, London, 1998)

Compared to the Victorian era, however, succinctness and understatement are in fashion:

> 'Life is short but love is long.'
> (Epitaph for 11-year-old boy, Mells churchyard, Somerset, 1960)

Similar sentiments are found in much greater quantity among 'in memoriam' columns in local newspapers. Their proprietors do not set themselves up as arbiters of taste in the way some clergy and cemetery authorities do, knowing perhaps the ephemeral nature of newsprint compared to carved granite:

> Though absent you are always near.
> Still loved and missed and very dear.
> (on third anniversary)

> My thoughts are always with you,
> my memories will never fade,
> I treasured all the years we shared
> and all the love you gave.
> (on fourth anniversary)

> Dad we love you more than words can say,
> and memories of you help us through each day,
> your help and advice always true.
> Oh Dad, how we miss you.
> (All three quotes from *Wiltshire & Gloucestershire*
> *Standard*, 11 February, 1999)

The stylized verses (Davies 1996) bring to public notice a remembrance that has remained private in the intervening months. In some communities, 'in memoriam' notices may be almost a social requirement, akin to Victorian high mourning, even if in private, the dead have been largely forgotten. The protestations of undying love in some notices may mask a highly ambivalent relationship. Research has yet to be done into the relationship between private feeling and public show, or mapping the social and geographical location of such columns and variations in their contents. Such research would tell us which of the peacetime dead are publicly remembered, where, and for how long.

Popular song sets similar verses to music. The sentiment 'You're mine for ever, baby' does not end at death. Just as in grand opera, the single most popular theme for pop song lyrics still concerns the love of boy and girl, so it should not be surprising that tragic death of the young lover is regularly found in popular song (Clayson 1997). Accidental death of the young blood hot-rodding it up Main Street, USA, was a particularly popular topic in lyrics of the 1960s, reflecting the very high rate of teenage fatalities before Ralph Nader's reforms to auto design took effect. Bikers also featured, as in 'Leader of the Pack'. More recently we have Eric Clapton's 'Tears from Heaven' about the accidental death of his 4-year-old son, and the best selling pop song of all time, Elton John's 1997 version of 'Candle in the Wind', saying goodbye to Princess Diana and assuring her that her legend will live for ever. Puff Daddy's 'Every Step I Take' followed soon after, remembering his murdered music partner; one worker with bereaved children told me they continually played this piece that expressed their sense of a continuing bond with those they had lost. Critics may dismiss much of this music as sentimental schmaltz, but no history of the popular culture of twentieth-century grief can afford to ignore it.

Moving to the other end of the age spectrum, Rory Williams' study of older Aberdonians includes a valuable chapter on bereavement in which he discusses (1990: 132–8) the tension between the irreplaceability of the deceased spouse and the need to replace him or her – if not through remarriage (unlikely for most older women) then through the society of widows and other sources of practical and emotional help. Williams found that the irretrievable nature of the loss was so taken for granted that it was rarely spoken of – except when attempts at replacement were made, in order presumably to reassure speaker and audience that this did not constitute a betrayal of the marriage. Bonds of loyalty to the dead had to be affirmed precisely because replacements were being sought. Those who remarried spoke of their new marriage as merely companionship, not the same as the marriage from which their family sprang.

Shapiro (1994: 11) describes a young North American widow with young children who appreciated going back to work: 'Because her family life, always a source of great joy and pleasure, now also served as a constant reminder of her grief and loss, she valued the new demands and relationships that came with her job, which allowed her to leave her grief momentarily behind her.' This woman oscillated between remembering and forgetting, between the world of the dead and the world of the living, between grief and a new role (compare Stroebe and Schut 1999). Shapiro notes (1994: 14) that children typically oscillate between forgetting and remembering: 'For children, the unremitting pace of adult grief is too intense, too much an interference with the necessary work of growing up. Children are more likely to put their grief down and pick it up again.' Elsewhere, however, Shapiro (1996: 323–5) provides a case study of a father who lost his favourite son and ended up leaving the family he loved, knowing that if he stayed in this world full of reminders of the dead he would have committed suicide. He was unable to oscillate between remembering and forgetting, and tragically had to abandon his family in order to forget.

It seems to me that (in Britain at least) the bystanders, those not themselves intimately bereaved but supporting the one who is, on the whole do not mind whether the bereaved person remembers or forgets. What they want is that the bereaved return as soon as possible to some kind of emotional stability, whether that involves remembering or forgetting. Both the bereaved person who is upset for months and years, and the one who never shows any upset, can be a worry and a burden. Those who show their grief but then soon get themselves together, or give a public appearance of such, are the least bother to others. No one, least of all the bereaved person, wants to be a bother to others, and being an emotional mess causes bother, as well as being painful both to experience and to behold. Bereavement counselling, typically motivated by the desire to ease suffering, can be appreciated by all concerned if it gets the emotions stabilized.

This is not to deny that there are subcultures in Britain or America where the peacetime dead are communally remembered. One is The Compassionate Friends, in whose local groups the members' dead children have a communal presence (see Chapter 11). Another is the Names Quilt, began in San Francisco in 1987 by gays, lesbians and their friends to commemorate those of their number who had died of AIDS. Each creatively embroidered panel commemorates an individual, yet laid out in settings such as the Mall in Washington DC, the thousands of panels comprising the quilt make a political statement of gay rights and the need to take AIDS seriously, as well as a focus of grief for individual family and friends. The dead are pressed into the service of creating solidarity both within the gay community, and between it and the straight community.

Anthropologist Nigel Barley (1995) has wittily observed that each academic discipline creates its own ancestors, who play a somewhat similar Durkheimian function to the AIDS quilt; that is, they help to define the group, in this case the discipline. How would we know what sociology was if sociologists did not pay homage to its founding fathers, Marx, Durkheim and Weber? What would philosophy be without Aristotle, Socrates and Plato, or physics without Newton, Faraday and Einstein? Any first year sociology student who has had to write an essay on Weber or Marx knows a little of what it is to revere the ancestors. Like members of many traditional societies, students may resent having to engage in this ritual, but engage in it they must: it has little to do with personal preference and everything to do with group identity.

Popular mourning of the deaths of the famous can also generate communal remembering. The immediate transformation of Diana Princess of Wales's memory into a cult resembling that of a medieval saint indicates that, in certain circumstances, popular culture – even in secular, historically Protestant Britain – can incorporate the dead. It is worth recalling (Cannadine 1981: 219–26) that the demand for a permanent memorial to the unknown soldier at the Cenotaph in Whitehall came from the popular enthusiasm for the temporary plaster memorial placed there by officialdom in 1919.

On the whole, though, it is only the war dead and the famous dead who are communally remembered. The more ordinary dead are like the more ordinary living: private individuals with whom society can dispense. Without a religious culture (as in Japan) or a popular culture (as in Victorian Britain) that encourages remembrance of the ordinary dead, they become just private memories in the hearts of those few to whom they were close.

Summary

This chapter outlined the historical development of grief and mourning in the twentieth century, focusing on the question of continuing versus breaking bonds with the dead. First, I looked at war and three responses to stress and loss that war has induced: forgetting, remembering and a confused inability to do either with any kind of balance. Second, I looked at peace, especially the effect of religious decline, the effect of palliative care and euthanasia, and the ambivalence between remembering and forgetting that seems to characterize many westerners at the end of the century. For the civilian dead, forgetting has dominated over remembering, at least in public.

Further reading

Bender, M.P. (1997) Bitter harvest: the implications of continuing war-related stress on reminiscence theory and practice. *Ageing and Society*, 17: 337–48.

Cannadine, D. (1981) War and death, grief and mourning in modern Britain, in J. Whaley (ed.) *Mirrors of Mortality: Studies in the Social History of Death*. London: Europa.

Mulkay, M. (1993) Social death in Britain, in D. Clark (ed.) *The Sociology of Death*. Oxford: Blackwell.

Winter, J. (1995) *Sites of Memory, Sites of Mourning: The Great War in European Cultural History*. Cambridge: Cambridge University Press.

Questions

1 'The dead are banished . . . never before have humans been able to kill so many people so efficiently or to forget them so completely.' Is Geary's (1994: 1–2) depiction of the twentieth century correct, or oversimplified?
2 'The decline of elaborate, stylized mourning rituals, which so success- fully cut off the bereaved from life-enhancing society, may actually make it easier for those who mourn to come to terms with their grief, as the demands of ordinary, daily life encourage them to pick up the threads once more.' (Cannadine 1981: 240) Do you agree?
3 If forgetting is how many (especially older) people cope with long-ago trauma, whether the trauma be of battle or of child abuse, it must be respected. Do you agree?
4 What do you believe about life after death?
5 Would you prefer to be buried or cremated, and why?

Notes

1 This observation was made at the Mind and Mortality conference, London, 19 March 1997.
2 Klass (1997: 172) argues that in the USA, as social cohesion diminishes, the war dead are decreasingly remembered. This does not appear to be occurring in the UK, despite (arguably) a similar decline in social cohesion.
3 Wilkinson (1978), however, argues that the established Anglican church was largely out of touch with the experiences of men at the front.

3 Private bonds

Contemporary western cultures do not make it easy for the non-famous peacetime dead to become communal ancestors, so what happens in the more private lives of bereaved people? Do they accept advice to let go, to forget, to move on? Or do they have their own private bonds with the dead? The answer is that some do and some do not. Some maintain a bond with the dead *and* move on to new relationships.

Some memories of the dead, such as sensing their presence, may come unbidden. Others thrive as a result of what Unruh (1983) terms 'strategic social action' – setting up a memorial, visiting a grave, visiting a place associated with the deceased. In this chapter, I review what is known about how individuals keep in touch with their dead and how they experience the dead keeping in touch with them. I look at four ways of keeping in touch: sensing the presence of the deceased, spiritual relationships with the dead, talking to the dead and rituals concerning particular artefacts and places. All four are illustrated in Winter's account of Käthe Kollwitz, the German artist and sculptress whose soldier son died in October 1914:

> In October 1916 she wrote in her diary that 'I can feel Peter's being. He consoles me, he helps me in my work.' She rejected the idea of spirits returning, but was drawn to the 'possibility of establishing a connection here, in this life of the sense, between the physically alive person and the essence of someone physically dead'. Call it 'theosophy or spiritism or mysticism', if you will, she noted, but the truth was there nonetheless. 'I have felt you, my boy – Oh, many, many times.' Even after the pain of loss began to fade, she still spoke to her dead son, especially when working on his memorial.
>
> (Winter 1995: 110)

In the next chapter, I look at how the dead can also be kept alive by their inclusion in conversations among the living.

Sensing the presence of the dead

The frequency with which bereaved people report sensing the presence of the dead was first researched by the Welsh physician, Dewi Rees (1971). Rees found that about half of widows and widowers had a sense of the presence of their dead spouse and that this was unrelated to gender, nationality, social class or social isolation. The experience was likely to take place at home and while awake. Three-quarters had never mentioned their experience to anyone else. Subsequent work has replicated his findings in a number of settings, summarized by Rees (1997: ch.17). The majority of these encounters are experienced as comforting and, though they tend to decline over time, there are plenty of examples of the dead appearing to comfort well-adjusted individuals decades later. The researcher is typically the first person spoken to about the experience, although some women may have confided it, hesitatingly, to one other woman friend. These are private experiences that may not easily be spoken of in a secular, historically Protestant culture, although with an increasing number of publications now documenting such experiences this may be beginning to change.

Though Rees himself paid proper respect to this phenomenon, it is significant that in his original work he (like many subsequent researchers) referred to 'hallucinations' and that the advisers for his PhD were psychiatrists. Many subsequent researchers, for example Parkes (1972), have also used this term. The word 'hallucination' is of recent Euro-American invention and no self-respecting anthropologist or student of comparative religion would use it to refer to experiences of the other world reported by non-western peoples. My dictionary defines 'hallucination' as an 'apparent perception of an object not present', so Rees was making a secularist assumption that the dead people being sensed were not actually there. It is a sign of a more developed phenomenological approach that is open to a variety of religious experience that Rees (1997) has now dropped the term and refers instead to 'continuing relationships with the dead'.[1] But we have yet to understand the importance of sensing the dead in sustaining the bond with the dead and how interactions with the dead compare with other experiences deemed hallucinatory (Bentall 1990).

Spiritual relationships

I have mentioned that a substantial number of elderly people in Britain believe that they will be reunited with their loved ones in the next life. For some, this translates into a desire to die sooner, in order to be with their pre-deceased spouse or child. If associated with depression, reluctance to eat or physical deterioration, this may be seen as a problem by carers, but student nurse Clare Pike (1983) questions this. She describes hospitalized 85-year-old Annie who went downhill after the death of the husband to whom she had been married for 60 years and who herself died on the day of his funeral. Rather than striving to boost Annie's morale and keep her alive, Pike asks if perhaps the nurses should have more positively accepted her wish to join her husband. Though from a nursing point of view, she was going 'downhill', from Annie's own viewpoint she was on her way 'uphill' to heaven. Michael Young raises the same issue. The mortality rates of widows and widowers in the first year after death are way above those for the still married, which is typically seen as a medical problem with articles documenting this typically being published in medical journals. But if the death of the first spouse creates great distress for the remaining spouse, the death of the second resolves it: 'One death may well cause another; a death can also cancel another' (Young and Cullen 1996: 181).

Afterlife beliefs of this kind are much less commonly held among younger age groups in Britain (Walter 1996a: 39–43), but in the more religious United States of America they are common. Nancy Hogan has studied the experiences of adolescents who lose a sibling, following deaths that can often be particularly traumatic such as car crashes and suicide. She identified 'vulnerable survivors' who struggle to find meaning in loss, whereas 'resilient survivors' find meaning in suffering. For several of the resilient survivors, this was found in future reunion and typically came after, rather than instead of, acceptance of the reality of the death.

> The acceptance of the impossibility of life as it was frees the energy of the bereaved siblings to reformulate a reality that includes the spiritual presence of their deceased siblings. It is the possibility of reunion in heaven/afterlife that begins the process of lessening the intensity of grief and that revitalizes the bereaved adolescents' sense of hope.
>
> (Hogan and DeSantis 1996: 250. See also Balk and Hogan 1995)

This creates a special sense of time that seems to me similar to the 'eternity' found in mystical religious experience. Living in the spiritual presence of the dead links not just heaven and earth, but past, present and future, dissolving temporal as well as spatial boundaries:

> The bereaved siblings learn to live with the physical absence and the simultaneous emotional presence of their deceased brother or sister. At the same time, the surviving siblings are anticipating a physical and social reunion in heaven with their deceased sibling. The simultaneous interaction of the phenomena of timelessness and ongoing attachment results in a sense of 'everywhen', a sense in which the past, present, and future are blended into a oneness.
>
> (Hogan and DeSantis 1992: 174)

Helen Elder, a British fourteen-year-old who lost her older sister Kate, later wrote about the spiritual comfort she found at the time. With religious teaching having very little influence on young people in Britain, and being herself neither religious nor belonging to a religious family, it is perhaps not surprising that the belief she describes is personal and intuitive, rather than doctrinally orthodox:

> What I had decided was not a religious revelation to me, it was a Helen belief, a personal belief, and the more I thought about it, the more I decided that Kate was definitely 'in the sky'. I was reluctant to call it heaven because of its religious connotation, and this new idea was very comforting. To me she was not lying six foot under the ground, but above me in the sunshine and the warm breezes and in the clouds.
>
> (Elder 1998: 127)

Another agnostic, seeing a close (and very religious) friend dead on her hospice bed had – and still has some years later – a powerful feeling that she is with the God he does not otherwise believe in. How many non-religious bereaved people in Britain create for themselves spiritual imagery of this kind is unknown. Chambers's (1997) study of religion in the Welsh town of Swansea found a number of women who had lost children and, in a culture of traditional gender roles, could not talk to their husbands, but could and did talk to God. The role of prayer in bereavement is distinctly under-researched.

Anecdotal evidence indicates that many bereaved people in Britain, particularly bereaved parents, consult spiritualist mediums in order to find out whether the loved one is all right. One middle-class woman told me about the unhappy life her mother had led and the tortuous relationship between mother and daughter. After her mother's death, she wanted to know her mother was at peace, and to this end – not knowing how otherwise to find a medium – visited a spiritualist church. With high levels of guilt and 'unfinished business', the daughter would have needed several sessions had she gone for therapy, but all she needed from the spiritualists was the assurance that her mother was at peace, an assurance she indeed received. She needed to know not about herself (the realm of therapy), but about the dead (the realm of certain forms of religion). Presumably, more conventional religious assurances that the deceased is at rest, and that both deceased and bereaved are forgiven, may have a similar effect for those who believe.

There are no figures indicating how many bereaved people consult mediums; the use they make of mediums is even less researched than is their use of prayer. Anecdotal evidence suggests that many bereaved people who consult a medium do so only once. Is this in fact typically the case? And if it is, is it because one consultation is effective, or is it sometimes because one consultation is ineffective? Or is it that the client recognizes its limited effectiveness and turns back to other friends or counsellors for further help? We simply do not know.

Whatever, I hope to have demonstrated in this section the possibility of recovering a place for the spiritual in the study and care of bereavement. Spiritual care has for some time been an accepted part of palliative care of the dying, yet has been markedly absent from bereavement care. That said, the spiritual in palliative care has largely turned away from traditional concerns about the next life to a broader concern with the patient's 'search for meaning' irrespective of whether this includes the next world (Walter 1997b). Understanding the spiritual meaning of bereavement, however, has to take seriously the afterlife, relationships with the dead, the supernatural, and both official and folk religious traditions.

Talking to the dead

In life, intimate relationships are developed and sustained through physical contact and through everyday conversation (Berger and Kellner 1964; Duck 1994). If relationships are to continue after death, we might expect to find not only a sense of physical presence, but also an ongoing conversation with the dead.

Little research has been done into the extent to which people talk to the dead. In Shuchter and Zisook's study of San Diego widows and widowers (1993: 34–5), over a third said they talked regularly with the deceased, a proportion declining only very slightly in the 13 months since the death. Another study found the cemetery to be a common place for adult children to talk to their dead parents:

> A 12-year-old girl whose mother died said 'I go to the cemetery when I feel sad and I need someone to talk with. Going to the cemetery makes me feel close.' A 15-year-old boy passed the cemetery on the way home from school: 'I don't talk about it much, but I stop by to visit about once a week. I tell him about my day and things I've done.'
> (Silverman and Nickman 1996: 79)

A BBC TV documentary, in which I participated, filmed one man whose son had died at the age of nineteen years and who regularly popped into the cemetery on his way to work 'to have a chat with the lad'. Other anecdotal examples abound of graveside conversations with the dead.

Cemetery behaviour, however, has only recently been systematically documented – by Doris Francis and her colleagues in a valuable ethnography in London. (This is one of very few participant observation studies of the social world of bereaved people, a gap in bereavement research in the modern West. Ethnographies are plentiful in traditional societies, but western studies of grief have relied overwhelmingly on interviews and questionnaires.)

Francis and co-workers found that men were particularly likely to come to the cemetery to have a chat:

> Middle age is a time when parents die. For many men, the cemetery offers a unique link with their dads. Occasionally on a quiet day, we will come upon a young man, almost invisible, as he kneels down planting or arranging flowers in front of his father's grave.
>
> Men come to the cemetery when things are not going well: a divorce or a broken relationship, a difficult time at work, a realisation that the father is gone and there was never enough time to talk and to get his needed guidance for life.
>
> There appear to be definite rules guiding these 'conversations' between father and son. The man must be alone and there should be no-one tending graves close by. Under such conditions, often while cleaning the stone or planting flowers, there is an openness in their 'conversations' which they never experienced when the parent was alive.
>
> (Francis *et al.* 1997: 18)

Those who have lost a spouse may regularly talk with the departed, telling them about family events such as the birth of a new grandchild or recalling memories of things done together (Francis *et al.* 1997: 20). Some of these grave-side encounters seek moral guidance from the dead, others help the bereaved person work out issues of self- and family identity, others simply continue the conversation that had been the bread and butter of the marital relationship, or create the conversation that sadly never existed between father and son.

Apart from cemeteries, important sites for these conversations have yet to be systematically researched. Women are more likely to sense the presence of the dead within the family home (Bennett 1987; Rees 1997) and they may be most likely to talk to them here. One experienced counsellor told me that many of her clients regularly talk with their dead children while alone driving the car; some admit to crying while driving and deliberately risking their lives, almost hoping for a crash that will take them from this life to join their children. Driving is private, and dangerous; a peculiarly modern link between this world and the next.

Symbolic places and things

As grave-side behaviour demonstrates, particular places can have a power to evoke the bond with the dead. This is clearly true of graves, shrines and memorials specifically set up to memorialize the dead. Edward Bailey, an Anglican priest and skilled observer of what he terms 'implicit religion', notes that in the average week more parishioners visit the churchyard in which their relatives are buried than actually enter his church for religious services. Indeed, he argues that the churchyard is not sanctified by the church, rather it is the other way around: the special affection the church building holds in the hearts of English villagers derives from its being surrounded by the village's dead.

Seeing and touching for the first time the name on the distant war grave of the father they never knew can be a profoundly important moment for adult children, thereby making his existence real (Walter 1993b). The Vietnam Memorial in Washington sees such reunions every day, often recorded in letters left there:

> Dad
> I came to visit you today. I haven't ever felt so close to you before. I never got a chance to know you but I love you very much. There isn't a day go by Mom doesn't think of you. Me and Gladene are always thinking of you too. You're gone from us now but we'll all be together again one day. You'll never be forgotten, you still live in every one of us. I'm really proud to be your son, I hope I can be as good a man as you were. I love you Dad and I'll be back to see you if its the last thing I ever do.
> Your son,
> Carwain L. Herrington, USN
>
> (Palmer 1988: 9)

If for westerners the grave or stone memorial is where the dead may be encountered, for contemporary Japanese it is the family altar, maintained even by some with otherwise no religion.

> The family altar would be your 'hot line'. As such, you could immediately ring the bell, light incense, and talk over the current crisis with one whom you have loved and cherished. When you were happy, you could smile and share your good feelings with him. When you were sad your tears would be in his presence. With all those who shared the grief he can be cherished, fed, berated, and idealised, and the relationship would be continuous from the live object to the revered ancestor ... The photograph of the deceased, the urn of ashes, the flowers, water, rice, and other offerings were all for the ancestor.
>
> (Yamamoto et al. 1969: 1663–4)

By bringing the shrine into the home, the Japanese combine what for many westerners are separated: the grave in a public place and sensing the presence of the dead among the familiar objects of home. There is therefore a particularly intense bonding with the dead at the Japanese shrine, but otherwise the feelings and behaviours seem not so different from those described above for westerners.

In the western home, photographs are a powerful locus of remembrance. Most households have scores if not hundreds of photos of members, especially children, snapped in everyday situations, on holiday, at extended family gatherings and celebrations, at birthdays and of children at play, in addition to formal photographs of children provided by their school. As one who grew up in the age of the light, cheap and easy-to-use camera, I find it hard to envisage what bereavement would be like without photographs (Riches and Dawson 1998a). Photographs, unlike letters and diaries, can be passed around a group and looked at by more than one person at a time, prompting the sharing of memories. People rarely look at family photos together without sharing memories. Videos are even more likely to be viewed communally, but perhaps offer less scope for reminiscence as a decision has to be made to pause the video in order to allow for talk.

Photographs of the dead have a long history. In the nineteenth century, when few households owned a camera and snapshots could not be taken of family members in natural postures, especially if they were moving, people turned after death to professional photographers to provide a memento. Burns (1990) provides a remarkable record of this tradition of post-mortem photography in America (where it may have flourished more than in Britain), with the dead propped up in a posture reminiscent of their former identity. Mid-century captions include 'Man sitting in a chair with a book' (1849), 'Older girl seated on love seat' (1852), 'Mother and father with dead daughter, useless medicine bottles on table' (1848). By the end of the century, the fashion turned toward depicting the dead sleeping in a silk-lined and flower-bedecked casket, foreshadowing the contemporary American wake: 'Johnny Frederick Schultz in white jewel box casket' (1893), 'Sleeping beauty under canopy in slumber room' (1915). In the twentieth century, large numbers of households have come to possess their own cameras, and with the decline in infant deaths even those who did not have a camera were more likely to have had professional photographs taken long before the death. Meanwhile, a norm seems to have arisen that photographing the dead is in bad taste. Nevertheless, there is evidence that, in the USA at least, photographing the dead continued, but was done privately by a family member (Ruby 1995). (Whether this private practice developed in the UK, where funeral directors provide less opportunity for viewing an embalmed and cosmeticized body, I do not know.) At the end of the twentieth century, however, a new tradition of publicly-legitimated post-mortem photography has been established in the UK, with maternity unit staff offering to provide parents with Instamatic photos of stillborn infants. Giving the child a name, a grave and keeping a lock of hair, also provide concrete evidence of the baby's existence, sex and appearance.

Any number of other objects can provide a link with the dead. Following Goffman (1959), Unruh (1983) writes about how in life we use props (clothes, consumer purchases, furniture, CDs, etc) as an 'identity kit' that fosters the impression of the identity we wish to present to both self and others. When we die, many of these props continue. Some may be kept by relatives as a memento. I, for example, have a clock that belonged to my grandfather, a coffee table that belonged to a much loved neighbour and a jacket that my father wore, and I chose each of them not only because they are useful but also because they have a story to tell. Unruh points out that before death we may specify that particular artefacts should pass on to particular people, thus ensuring some control over our post-mortem identity. We may destroy other things, such as embarrassing or incriminating letters, before our deaths, for the same reason. In the British television *Antiques Roadshow* people bring antiques, a vase or a watch or whatever, to be valued by experts, and in the process talk about the circumstances surrounding the object, how it came to be in the family and so forth; such objects, along with talking about them, are links with the family's past and with the ancestors (Radley 1990).[2]

Artefacts can trigger cherished memories, and can be deliberately sought. Parkes (1986: 70–1) found that half the London widows he interviewed felt drawn to places associated with their husbands and most were reluctant to leave the home where they had lived, treasuring possessions and parts of the house that were especially 'his'. The smell of his clothes could also evoke his presence. But artefacts can also turn up unexpectedly, causing distress to bereaved people who wish to have some control over when they are, and when they are not, reminded of the deceased. They can also vanish unexpectedly. In the UK, so long as an inquest or criminal trial is still pending, the authorities can hold on to any of the deceased's possessions that may be needed as evidence in court. A suicide note, written for the family, becomes the property of the crown, and the family may not be aware they can ask for it back after the inquest (Biddle 1998). At the time of writing, ten years after the Lockerbie disaster, relatives still await the return of their loved one's possessions. Relatives may feel that until such possessions are indeed within their possession, the deceased is not yet truly theirs.

Functions

What functions do the various contacts with the dead described in this chapter play for bereaved people? Different theories of bereavement (see Chapter 6) suggest different answers to this question and I conclude this chapter by sketching the various positions.

One position is to take contacts with the dead at face value, namely that they do indeed represent the dead intervening in various ways to continue their support for those they love. This is the view of a number of religious people. The empirical social sciences can neither prove nor falsify this belief, and it is not their business to, though they can examine its consequences. I therefore look at theories that seek causes and consequences within this world.

First, there is the ethological framework developed by Bowlby (1980) and Parkes (1986). They argue that there is survival value in the young animal searching for the parent after accidental separation; through evolution, it has therefore become instinctual to seek any lost significant other. Parkes (1986: 60–96) thus explains sensing the presence of the dead and cherishing as 'searching' or 'pining' for the deceased. Eventually proving unsuccessful, it may help mourners confirm for themselves the reality that they are now on their own; this explains why sensing the presence of the dead tends to decrease in frequency over time. Parkes (1986: 79–80) adds that 'as time passes, if all goes well, the intensity of pining diminishes and the pain of pining and the pleasure of recollection are experienced as a bitter-sweet mixture of emotions, nostalgia'. Rees (1997: 202) is sceptical of this explanation of the sense of presence, because (1) the sense is not usually initiated by the living, (2) it does not match other searching behaviour in which people know exactly what they are looking for, and (3) it is by no means uncommon years after the loss. Rees admits, however, that the sense of presence does, on average, decrease with time.

Second, Rosenblatt's reminder theory (Rosenblatt *et al.* 1976; Rosenblatt 1983; introduced on page 27 of this book) and Stroebe's dual process or oscillation theory (Stroebe and Schut 1999) both indicate how many people value a combination of contacts with the dead and getting on without them. There is no necessary direction to this and it is likely to continue indefinitely. From his study of nineteenth-century diaries, Rosenblatt argues that the sense of presence, spiritualism, prayer, hope of reunion and using the deceased's wishes as a moral guide can all be seen as attempts to resist change (compare Marris 1974). Paradoxically, such attempts may actually promote change:

> Dreams of the lost and the sense of his or her presence tell one that the lost is actually gone . . . The process of communicating through a medium . . . apparently cannot be sustained . . . and alters the relationship. Prayer to the lost tends to deal only with the spiritual area, in which the risk of being rejected by the lost person is relatively slight . . . Planning to reunite with a deceased person also seems to reflect the awareness of change, since the plans reported in the diaries never included mundane content.
>
> (Rosenblatt 1983: 149)

Such contacts, while enabling the bond to persist, also remind the mourner that the dead are dead, rendering the physical loss all too real. As a Japanese widow reported (Yamamoto *et al.* 1969: 1664) 'When I look at his smiling face (in his photo), I feel he is alive, but then I look at the urn and know he is dead.' So, contra Parkes, contacts with the dead need not represent searching, and need not diminish over time, but – and here we may agree with Parkes – they do function to confirm the reality of death.

A third view is that there is less a letting go of the dead person than a letting go of uncomfortable feelings such as anger and guilt. Once these are gone, it becomes possible to remember the deceased with pleasurable feelings and to internalize them (Rubin 1984). Four years after her sister Kate's death, during which she experienced shock, severe depression and suicidal thoughts of joining her, Alex Elder wrote:

> But I will live to tell your tale
> you will remain within my heart for all my days
> I will strive, fight,
> love, laugh,
> with you beside me.
> We will march through life together
> strong

(Elder 1998: 135)

With the dead safely internalized, sensing their presence, visits to the grave and cherishing objects and memories can continue indefinitely, or may even increase over time. Or they may no longer be necessary. As the shock of the death, and also perhaps bad memories of the actual death, wear off, so it becomes possible to recall with pleasure the person in the many years before. Alex recalls the day when she looked at a photo of Kate and did not cry, but smiled instead. For widows, Jane Littlewood has described this as 'falling in love backwards' – at first you are too shocked to remember much, but with time you begin to recall and enjoy more and more memories. This is Parkes's bitter-sweet nostalgia. As one of the widows interviewed by Parkes (1972: 104) put it, when asked whether she felt her husband's presence: 'It's not a sense of his presence, he's here inside me. That's why I'm happy all the time. It's as if two people are one . . . although I'm alone, we're sort of together if you see what I mean.' (See also Marris 1974: 37–38.)

Fourth, Marwit and Klass (1995) asked a sample of students aged 18–54 years to identify and write about an important person in their lives who had died, looking in particular at the role (if any) the deceased currently played in their life. The deaths were of grandparents, peers and older friends, with only one participant each describing the death of a father, aunt, uncle or spouse. No participant had trouble with the concept and many wrote two to three pages. Four kinds of role played by the deceased were identified: role model, giving guidance in specific situations, clarifying the values of the survivor and as a valued part of the survivor's biography. Though this is as yet only conjecture, we may ask whether Marwit and Klass's finding may be linked to the data on contacting the dead. Is one consequence of sensing, talking to, praying for the dead that they become more real to the bereaved as role models, providers of guidance and as clarifiers of values? We certainly know that people who talk to the dead often ask for guidance or clarification.

An example of how experiencing the dead can lead to their becoming an inspirational role model is found in the song 'Joe Hill', recorded on disc by Paul Robeson. Joe is a working man shot for a murder he did not commit and whom ten years later the singer is surprised to meet. The singer is reassured by Joe that he never died and by the end of the song the message is clear: wherever working men are fighting for their rights, there Joe is.

Fifth, Walter (1996b) has highlighted Marwit and Klass's final role for the dead, namely their being a valued part of the survivor's biography. Finding out who the deceased was may be important for finding out who I am, though it seems likely that this will be assisted less by the private encounters with the dead described in this chapter and more by the conversations with the living to be described in the next chapter.

Summary

In contemporary western societies in which ancestors are not, generally, publicly remembered, the dead live on, if at all, in more private ways. This chapter has examined four of the chief ways in which this happens: (1) through sensing the presence of the dead; (2) through religious beliefs and consulting spiritualist mediums; (3) through talking to the dead (not least at the grave-side); and (4) through linking objects such as the grave, family altar, photographs and other mementoes. How we analyse these experiences depends on our theory of bereavement and the chapter concludes with a number of interpretations.

Further reading

Klass, D., Silverman, P.R. and Nickman, S.L. (eds) (1996) *Continuing Bonds: New Understandings of Grief*. Bristol, PA and London: Taylor & Francis.

Rees, D. (1997) *Death and Bereavement: The Psychological, Religious and Cultural Interfaces*. London: Whurr.

Unruh, D. (1983) Death and personal history: strategies of identity preservation. *Social Problems*, 30(3): 340–51.

Questions

1 Do you relate to the dead in any of the ways described in this chapter?
2 Do you agree that it is inappropriate to describe sensing the presence of the dead as a 'hallucination'?

3 Which of the five functions played by contacts with the dead (as described in the last section) do you find most plausible, and why?

Notes

1 My position here is methodological agnosticism. In social science research, we cannot assume that God, or contacts with the dead, really do exist; and we cannot assume that they really do not exist. But we have to take seriously what bereaved people say, whether or not their beliefs and experiences are ones we can personally share. I presume that counsellors and therapists normally remain similarly agnostic in their work.
2 I am indebted to Sheila Payne for this observation.

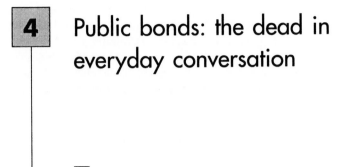

4 Public bonds: the dead in everyday conversation

For a deceased person in the West today who is mourned by more than one rememberer, there is comparatively little provision for the mutual interplay of their memories of him.

(Vitebsky 1993: 259)

Call me by my old familiar name,
speak to me in the easy way you always used . . .
Let my name be ever the household word it always was.

(Henry Scott Holland)

That families often ask that Scott Holland's poem be read at funerals in the UK suggests that his sentiments resonate with a considerable number of bereaved Britons. Yet the quote from Vitebsky, an anthropologist commenting on the West from his perspective in India, suggests that in practice the deceased's name is by no means always the household word it always was. This chapter looks at the extent to which the dead live on through everyday conversation.

Theory

Why is this issue important? Four theoretical grounds may be stated. The first is that if I am to become an ancestor, to have some existence in the ongoing life of the group, then the group must continue to talk about me. If people no longer mention my name, I will be forgotten as far as communal memory is concerned and I will cease to exist as an ancestor. In traditional societies, this talk would be as likely to occur in specific rituals as much as in everyday conversation. The ritual acts of remembrance of Jews and Hindus, along with the ritualized grave-side visits of the rural Greeks described by Danforth (1982), all involve survivors talking about the one who has died. For those westerners who no longer have such religiously required rituals, the dead can still live on in communal memory, so long as the group continues to talk about them. Sharing of post-mortem reminiscences with other family members has been described by Rosenblatt and Elde (1990) and by Silverman and Nickman (1996) who emphasize how this helps individuals create their own personal construct of the deceased. This chapter examines how reminiscence creates a place for the dead in the life of groups as well as of individuals. It is not just that the group may help the grieving individual; the individual can help the grieving group.

Second, the importance of talk, not just about the dead, has been highlighted by Seale (1998) and Nadeau (1998). Seale combines Berger's (1969) argument that society is ultimately a defence against the chaos and anomie of death, with the insight of the ethnomethodologists (e.g. Sudnow 1967) that social order is created in the minutiae of everyday conversation. Thus, it is everyday conversation, of all kinds, that most of the time keeps at bay the existential threat posed by human mortality. Historically, religion and religious ritual have been central to how this has been achieved, but the more secular a society becomes the more the burden is placed on apparently banal everyday talk. The appearance of the dead in everyday conversation may therefore affect how survivors cope. Indeed, one of the most frequent complaints from bereaved people is that others get the conversation wrong: 'my son won't ever mention his father', 'I wish mum wouldn't keep mentioning dad', 'they don't know how to talk to me, I have to take the initiative' and, of course, the proverbial 'they cross to the other side of the street to avoid having to speak to me'.

Third, bereavement (whether through death, disability, unemployment, relationship break-up, or whatever) is the state of being caught between the present, a past and a lost future. Rewriting the past to make sense of the new present is crucial if sense is to be made of change and the future faced. Following Jerome Brunner, Frank (1995: 65) defines reflexivity as 'the perpetual readjustment of past and present to create and sustain a good story'. Telling the story of the lost one and how they were lost, going over it with others as well as in one's own head, is a typical experience of bereavement, especially if the death was unexpected. Only then can survivors begin to get a handle on their new situation. When the death is highly problematic, as with suicide or AIDS, the need to create a good enough story is paramount, yet it is often precisely with such stigmatized deaths that it may prove impossible to talk to others about what happened (see the next chapter). Mutual help bereavement groups (Chapter 11) can be valued by survivors precisely because they allow them to tell the stories others have not wanted to hear, or have tired of.

This process of storymaking has been described by Robert Weiss (1975) as it applies to marital separation (see also Harvey 1996: 11). Creating an account or story that makes sense of how the marriage broke up or why the partner left is important if the person is to organize their chaotic thoughts about why the marriage ended, if they are to sense they have some control over things and if they are to settle amicably the question of who is responsible for what. By creating a story about the marriage with a beginning, a middle and an end, some detachment from otherwise crippling emotions can be achieved. It seems that a similar process often occurs when someone is lost through death. Sometimes the bereaved person literally writes the story of the person's life and death, this being one sub-set of popular bereavement literature (see, for example, Koppelman's (1994) biography of his teenage son who died in a car crash).

Fourth, telling the dead person's story tells the storymaker who the deceased was, and by extension who the storymaker is (Walter 1996b). We create our selves through interacting with others, so it can be important, following a death, to know more about the one who has died. This may seem strange to some readers: surely a wife of 30 years knows pretty much all there is to be known about her husband? But in many bereavements, this is not so. Parents by no means know everything about their teenage children, especially what they get up to with their peers; Koppelman (1994) talked at length to his son's peers so that he could piece together his son's life. Parents of middle aged children who die may have grown apart from them. Children go through chests of old photos and letters to gain a fuller picture of their now deceased parents. Those who lost their parents through death or adoption when they were very little and who have no direct memories of them, may be intensely interested to know more about them (Nickman 1996). One humanist funeral officiant says that a quarter of the appreciative letters he has received from families refer not only to the funeral, but also to the pre-funeral meeting where they go through the person's life so that the officiant can construct a eulogy. For example, 'We didn't expect that simply reconstructing Bill's life, with all its troubles, would give us all a more understanding view of the difficulties we had with him.'

Because of the separation of home and work, the work lives of parent or spouse may be opaque to others in the family. When my father died, I found letters of condolence from his ex-colleagues of particular interest, helping me fill out my understanding of who he was, and hence of who I am. Finding out precisely who it was who brought me up, or who I was married to, or what became of my adolescent child, can be crucial to this project of discovering the self, whether done pre- or post-mortem.

Personal identity – who precisely I am – is a concern for many (Berger *et al.* 1974; Giddens 1991). In large scale urban societies, we inhabit varied and non-overlapping social worlds: the people I work with, commute with, play golf with, go to church with, live with are likely to be different groups.

I play different roles and take on different identities in each setting, so knowing who I 'really' am can become problematic. The most popular ways of resolving this are (1) to believe in a real, inner me that exists independent of the many and often conflicting roles I have to play, and (2) to join my real inner me with another real inner me, that is, to fall in love and set up house together (Berger and Kellner 1964). We can then together have children who in turn affirm the joint identity we have created within the marriage. In other words, we need marriage and the family in order to sustain the precarious sense of who we 'really' are. In practice, of course, we do not control our children totally and there may be chunks of our partner's life that are outwith our ken. Hence the importance on the death of a partner, parent or child of finding out who they were in order to find out who we are.

Even in an apparently good marriage, there may be much there is unknown about the partner. In Krzysztof Kieslowski's movie *Blue*, a young widow grieves deeply over the sudden death of her husband and son; life has no meaning, until she discovers by accident that he had been conducting an affair for many years. She totally re-writes the story of her marriage and hence of her present situation, enabling her to move out of her melancholy and start living and loving again. This indicates that the story may well change over time. 'The longer people are dead, the more your relationship with them changes' (Harvey 1996: 142).

Conversation partners: present or absent?

The most obvious conversation partners are usually others who knew the deceased, for it is in conversation with them that the deceased is most likely to feature. But many family and friendship groups in the contemporary West often are not able to speak of their dead, at least not on an everyday basis. This may be because cultural norms prevent it. In Britain, for example, though there is no rule that says one may not speak of the dead, there is a rule never to speak ill of them and many people are unwilling to mention the dead if they think this will upset either themselves or others (Gorer 1965). Since bereavement is an upsetting business and the dead are never perfect, this can considerably limit conversations about them! Many families experience such limitations (Shapiro 1994: 15). Because nobody in the family would talk about him, Laura Prince (1996) wrote a biographical book 25 years later about what happened after the death of her 13-year-old brother, Mathew. She called her book *Breaking the Silence*, the implication being that her family is a metaphor for a society that will not speak of the dead. Blank (1998: 36) and similarly bereaved parents have found that other parents do not like them talking about their dead child, as it brings to the surface every parent's worst fears for the safety of their own children.

We have already seen (page 20) that stepmothers may not like the children talking about their natural mother.

Even if culture and personal preference do allow the dead to be spoken of, social, geographical and family structure may hinder it. Others who knew the deceased may simply not be around. The dead cannot be included in everyday conversation if those who knew the dead do not live, work or socialize together, as is becoming increasingly common in westernized societies. This may be contrasted with stable small-scale communities in which those encountered daily by the mourner typically also knew the deceased, and where it is not hard (if cultural norms allow) for the deceased's name to live for a generation or two in everyday conversation. The structural factors limiting this in affluent western societies are social fragmentation, family fragmentation, geographical mobility and longevity.

Social fragmentation

I have noted above the way in which the modern urban person's social, work and family groups do not typically overlap. So, when a close family member dies, my colleagues at work are unlikely to have met her; likewise if a colleague drops dead at work, my family are unlikely to have known her. Colleagues or family can say 'I'm sorry', meaning they are sorry *for* me, but they are not themselves sorry, because they never knew the deceased. In totally anonymous settings, such as on public transport or in a shopping mall, nobody may be even aware I am bereaved, creating the painful sensation that the world is continuing as though nothing has happened. More than a few bereaved parents have wanted to scream out and tell strangers in the shopping mall 'My baby has died!' The very social fragmentation that makes personal identity problematic and that may underlie the need to talk to others about the deceased is precisely what makes it difficult finding others who knew the deceased. The same is true of the remaining three factors.

Family fragmentation

Fragmentation within the extended family is currently increasing. New family types, primarily reconstituted families (following divorce) and gay couples, can cause rifts between close kin. A child's grandad, his father's father, dies, but the child's absentee father has lost touch and the child's mother wants nothing to do with the father's family, which she feels sided with him against her in the divorce. The child is therefore isolated from his deceased grandfather's kin. Gay couples can also be cut off by rejection. A man in his 30s loses his partner through AIDS and the dead man's parents take over the funeral and the role of chief mourner (losing an adult child can be one of the most painful of losses), refusing to acknowledge their son's sexuality and refusing to acknowledge his partner. He and the parents cannot create a common biography of the dead man. This is not to say that the past never saw one part of an extended family refusing to speak to another, far from it, but the current rise of divorce and of homosexual partnerships certainly can have an impact on whether one bereaved person can share the deceased's story with another.

Longevity

The twentieth century is the first in western history in which the typical death is not that of a child. Most children reach adulthood, and most adults reach old age. So the most common death is in old age, long after the children have moved out, leaving a widow or widower on his or her own, and leaving adult children geographically separated both from the surviving parent and from each other. When the typical death was of a child, the chief mourners (parents, siblings) were usually co-resident; now the typical death is of an old person, the chief mourners (spouse, children) are usually living in separate homes and often in separate parts of the country.

Geographical mobility

Living away from kin is related to urbanism and to class (Fischer 1977) as well as to longevity, but the key factor is geographical mobility (Wenger 1995). The geographically mobile are those least likely to have daily face-to-face interactions with other family members who knew the deceased well. Not only do they live in separate homes, but their homes are distant from each other.

This last trend should not be exaggerated, because a fair amount of residential propinquity still exists. In the UK substantial proportions of elderly people live near to adult children (Warnes *et al.* 1985; Qureshi and Walker 1989; Wenger 1995), and in the USA the extended family can still be important, the telephone and the automobile shrinking geographical distance (Litwak 1965). The letter of condolence and the telephone keep bereaved people in touch with family and friends who knew the deceased. Rosenblatt and Elde (1990) found that all of their adult mid-Western respondents had reminisced with siblings about their deceased parent, though for several this was primarily when they got together for the funeral. Most bereaved people are elderly, and though the elderly widow is likely to live on her own she is likely to have regular – even if not daily – contact with kin, either face-to-face or on the phone. I have described elsewhere (Walter 1999a) how among the mobile, friends and neighbours may to some extent replace kin, and in some circumstances the death of a neighbour can become part of the street folklore, so that the person becomes a 'street ancestor' helping to create a street identity.

Nevertheless, the overall trend, taking all four factors into account, is that it is increasingly difficult for bereaved people together to construct the deceased as an honoured ancestor, except in highly private and individualized ways. The bond with the dead is continued internally within bereaved individuals: it is hard for the dead to be part of the social life of ongoing residential or work groups. The bereaved person is individuated out from the mass and is surrounded by people who did not know the deceased well, if at all, and do not share the pain. Everyday conversation becomes problematic.

This may shed some light on the question of grief's universality. Clearly all human beings grieve, but is there a universal 'grief process'? (Rosenblatt *et al.* 1976; Stroebe and Stroebe 1987: ch.3; Klass, forthcoming). If grief is defined in terms of feelings and mourning in terms of social behaviour, then an answer often given is that the feelings of grief are universal but they are expressed differently according to culture. This chapter suggests a somewhat different angle. If we look at bereavement in terms of loss by groups as well as by individuals, then it is clear that bereavement is a hugely different experience depending on whether the loss has been by a coherent group or by a few isolated individuals. If we see grief as involving not only emotions but also a story, an identity and an ancestor to be created, then it will vary enormously both across and within societies.

It should now be clear why, following a tragedy such as the untimely death of a national hero, colleague or schoolmate, there may be a reversion not only to more elaborate funeral rituals but also to a largely lost form of mourning. This is because those met in everyday life are also mourners. Talking about the dead becomes a routine matter. After the death of Diana, Princess of Wales, in 1997, many people were bemused by this, feeling they had to explain it in terms of the media constantly keeping her in the public eye or in terms of a change in national character. Though the media were indeed influential, one does not need this to explain the ongoing conversations about her. It is simply what normally happens when a group, rather than a scattering of isolated individuals, loses a member, especially if that member is royal, beautiful, powerful, controversial and dies in tragic circumstances. The same happened following the death of Princess Charlotte in 1817, long before the invention of television and the mass society (Schor 1994; Wolffe 1999).

Widowhood

There is evidence that bereaved persons who are socially isolated are likely to find life particularly hard (Clayton 1975) and there are several possible reasons for this (Rosenblatt 1983: 107–9). The person will not have enough distractions and may ruminate endlessly on the loss. Durkheim (1952) has argued that social isolation for anyone, bereaved or not, is associated with personal dissatisfaction. The thesis of this chapter points specifically to the isolated person's lack of anyone with whom to talk; there is nobody with whom to develop and edit the story of the deceased and what they meant to the survivor (Cochran and Claspell 1987). One function of counselling, not always fully recognized, is to help with editing the story when no one else is willing or able.

As we have seen, those living with others may nevertheless feel isolated if other members of the household cannot or will not speak of the dead. But the dangers of isolation do suggest that widow(er)hood when there are no co-resident children is a particular kind of bereavement, because the person's main conversation partner has been removed. It is the most common situation in which one loses not only someone much loved, but also one's main partner in conversation with whom one would otherwise discuss both the little things and the big things (such as bereavement). In so far as marriages are built up through everyday conversation, the widow or widower mourns the loss of the very conversation that had hitherto helped them repair life's stresses.

There is evidence that, in the USA at least, widowers tend to be more isolated than widows and that this may have consequences for their health (Ferraro *et al.* 1984). Women tend to talk more than do men about both intimate feelings and everyday events to their friends, which means that widows may find it easier than widowers to elaborate the story of their marriage with their friends. They may also be more able than males to talk to their children. That said, widows are more likely than widowers to be excluded from socializing with couples they had previously known as friends; somehow the widow, but not the widower, is perceived as a threat to the couple's marriage. Widows are more likely than widowers to have invested more of their identity in the marriage and may therefore be more bereft (Silverman 1986).

Widowers are more likely than widows to remarry. This is partly due to the greater availability of women, especially in the older age groups, but it may also have to do with the greater isolation felt by bereaved males and their greater willingness to see the wife as replaceable. Remarriage raises the question of whether the dead partner can be spoken of in the new marriage. The threat is revealed in Amado's novel (1968) *Dona Flor and Her Two Husbands*, subsequently made into a film, where a widow remarries while carrying on an affair with the ghost of her first husband. Moss and Moss (1996) describe remarriage following death as a triadic relationship in which there are three people, suggesting that the new partner who can accept the role of their spouse's dead partner is likely to enjoy a better marriage. I think of a young woman whose previous partner died and who is now remarried; he is often referred to and his parents play the role of grandparents to the children of her new marriage. Parkes (1998a), however, warns that the presence in a second marriage of an idealized first spouse can cause a widow to denigrate the new husband and undermine the new marriage.

Many second marriages, however, exclude the dead spouse. Some elderly British women wait till their second husband is dead before going on pilgrimage abroad to visit, for the first time, the grave of their first husband, killed in the Second World War. It may be, of course, that such a woman had been too busy caring for an ailing second husband to contemplate trekking off to Burma or North Africa. It may be, however, that the first husband – dying young and idealized by her – was too much of a threat to her second marriage. Or it may simply be that, like so many others, she had put the war and its traumas – including her husband's death – behind her, and only in the emptiness of second widowhood do her thoughts, prompted by the considerable publicity currently given to war grave pilgrimages, eventually return to her youth.

Student bereavement

I will briefly discuss one other kind of bereavement: that experienced by a student away at college. I have already mentioned this in a previous chapter in the context of oscillation between forgetting and remembering, but it can also be examined in terms of conversation partners. The student's life is split between half the year at college and half the year elsewhere, possibly at home. Whether the deceased is a fellow student or, more likely a relative, the student experiences two worlds: one in which the deceased played an important part, the other in which the deceased played no part whatsoever. The student may find that fellow students take little or no interest in their friend's dead grandfather whom they had never met and indeed of whose existence they had not previously been aware. Though college may be a blessed relief from the pall of grief at home (say if a grandparent had died), college can also be painful if nobody there wants to hear the story.

Every year one or two such students make their way to me as their tutor and seem to value just being able to talk about their relative. Being male, I am uneasy probing into their feelings, and female students are in any case better hugged by their best friend or boyfriend than by their male tutor, but my opening question 'Tell me about him/her' enables the student to tell the story, a story which incidentally may well be full of feeling. Little research has been conducted into this specific form of bereavement, still less into the role of storytelling within it. There are, of course, comparable bereavements, such as in the armed services and the merchant navy, where people work for months at a time in close collaboration with peers and away from the family home.

Practical implications

If this chapter is correct in identifying reflexive modern individuals' need, yet lack of opportunity, to talk about their dead, then this has implications for those who work with bereaved people. But first a caveat. Although I have outlined some good reasons why survivors include the dead in every-day conversation, there is no reason why everyone should, and many indeed wish to be more private with their memories (Elder 1998). There are wide variations in how people respond to bereavement and they are no more likely all to thrive on talking about the dead than they are to go through the stages of grief (Chapter 6) or to share their feelings (Chapter 9).

The funeral

Ideas that it is wrong to speak of the dead, or that people will necessarily be embarrassed by such speech, can be challenged by those who lead funerals, simply by speaking publicly about the dead with love, humour and honesty. The move toward funerals that celebrate a life is now well established, not only in secular and humanist (in Australia life-centred) funerals but also in many led by clergy. I have written at length elsewhere (Walter 1990) on how this may be done, emphasizing the need to do it well or not at all. Mourners typically value a funeral that captures the personality of the person who has died, through symbols and song as well as in words, so long as they can identify with the story told. Clergy or other celebrants can easily get the story wrong if they take too little care in preparation, or listen only to the idealized story provided by the next of kin, a story that bears little relation to the real person known by the variety of mourners present. It is precisely a person's failings that often make them loveable.[1]

The funeral that succeeds in telling the story and that shows how it is possible to speak with love about someone's failings, gives the mourners permission to elaborate the story further, not only at the social gathering following the funeral but in the weeks, months and years that follow. Elaborating the story together does not require any great skill; it is, after all, what mourners have done for millennia.

Memory books

The funeral, and subsequent religious rituals such as the Jewish *shiveh* and *yahrzeit*, are not the only ways in which the story can be ritually told. Memory books and books of remembrance are becoming popular in some organizations. The children's charity, Barnardo's, advertises its memory store and memory book as an aid both to acknowledging feelings and to telling the story:

After illness, death or divorce, it is all too easy to break the thread of the family's history, to lose important contacts and for children to be unsure about what really happened in the past. *Memory Store* and *Memory Book* are specially designed to help children facing family crisis. Here is a practical way to help children acknowledge feelings of loss and grief and to preserve vital information about their family identity . . . And when parents are no longer there to answer questions, the *Memory Book* helps children find out about their first words, how their name was chosen, the jokes and traditions that were special in their home.

If the story cannot be spoken, it can be written, even painted.

Mutual help groups

Even with encouragement, there may be no one willing or able to listen to, let alone elaborate, the story of the dead person. Mutual help groups, especially for those who have lost children, provide a setting in which the dead can be spoken of. Indeed, Klass's study (1988, 1997) of an American chapter of Bereaved Parents (formerly The Compassionate Friends) found that the dead children become central to the conversational life of the group and may gain a shared reality there that they are denied in conversation with those who actually knew them in life. Klass argues that this shared social reality helps each parent find a secure place for their child in their own heart.

Counselling

There is no comparable study showing whether this kind of process occurs in bereavement counselling, but it seems likely that for some clients it does. In my own workshops and lectures in which I have propounded a model of grief based on biographical reconstruction (Walter 1996b), counsellors have often told me that they do indeed encourage their clients to tell the story of the dead and of the death. Less directive counsellors say that the client often tells the story anyway (McLaren 1998). This may be particularly valued by the client if no one else is able or willing to participate in the storytelling – but this speculative statement needs to be researched.

Idealization

At this point, the question of idealization must be discussed. It is well known that survivors often idealize the dead: we tend to miss the good things about the person and to forget the bad. Many a dead husband is the best who ever lived, many a dead 2-year-old the most angelic. The counsellor may wish to respect this. One way of doing this is to put on the back burner the normal counselling ethos of empathy, which is based on an assumption of human commonality, and to put on the front burner an ethos of genuine interest in the deceased, which is based on an assumption of his or her being unique and special. This, rather than empathy, is the dominant attitude of a life-centred celebrant when conducting the pre-funeral interview with the family (Walter 1990: 218) and might also be appropriate to story-telling counselling sessions. Put another way, the celebrant is as interested in the deceased as in the survivor, as are the members of some mutual help groups, and counsellors too might consider this.[2]

Counselling can, however, find a role in challenging idealization. Indeed, some bereaved people go for counselling precisely because they cannot stand the idealization that is expected in the family. An adult daughter abused by her father may be distressed by her mother's portraying him as a paragon of virtue and may not have the heart or the courage to disillusion her. She may need to speak to a stranger about such matters, one skilled in helping her to handle painful memories. In this framework then, mutual help groups and counselling can help the person tell, elaborate and edit the deceased's story, or enable the person to develop a story that they can embrace. Chapter 11 explores this in more detail.

Need the story be true?

This brings us to the question of whether the story need be true. Narrative therapy (Spence 1982; Sarbin 1986b; McAdams 1993) would say not. Here the therapist sees the person as having many stories, none of which is the 'real' or 'underlying' story; the person is in difficulties because their dominant stories are unhelpful, portraying themselves as, for example, victims governed by fate. The aim of this kind of therapy is to promote hitherto minor stories that are more positive for the client.

This may be fine in one-to-one therapy governed by a norm of confidentiality, but it should be clear by now that the richest and often most sustaining stories told by survivors are those they can tell together. Many stories about the dead are public, and need to be seen to be true. South Africa's Truth and Reconciliation Commission is a case in point: people want to know the truth about how their relative died. Likewise, a funeral eulogy must be good enough to be recognized by a wide range of mourners. This is also true of published obituaries. An article in *The Independent* (7 March 1996) titled 'Peer's family attack offensive obituary' starts, 'The family of Lord Jay, who has died aged 88, last night defended the former Labour Cabinet minister against an obituary which claimed he was mean, shabby and mediocre.' Obituaries, like funeral eulogies, have to weave a story that is true enough to be recognized but not so negative as to be upsetting. Historical novelists and movie makers face a similar issue, as illustrated by an article titled 'A mistake of titanic proportions':

The makers of the film *Titanic* have apologised to a Scottish town for turning its local hero into a villain, a British member of parliament said yesterday. The Oscar-winning Hollywood movie showed the Titanic's first officer, William Murdoch, taking a bribe, shooting a third-class passenger who tried to fight his way into a lifeboat and then turning his gun on himself. 20th Century Fox admitted in a letter to Alisdair Morgan, the member of parliament for Murdoch's home town Dalbeattie, that it had no evidence that the first officer of the fated ship had done any of those things.

(*Cape Times* [South Africa] 9 April 1998)

In the year following her death, the press's repeated telling and retelling of the story of Diana, Princess of Wales, with some newspapers paying scant respect for hard evidence, may have been upsetting for her two teenage children. They might well prefer people would stop telling her story.

Within families, individual members may hold to different accounts of the deceased member only if they do not need to co-operate. But if two brothers wish to continue the family business 'the way dad would have wanted', they need to agree on what kind of person dad was and what he would have wanted. If a woman dies and her husband and mother are to co-operate in raising her children 'the way she would have wanted', then they must agree over who the dead woman was and what her ideas of child-rearing were. This can be particularly tricky if the mother knew her from ages 0–18, and the husband from ages 30–40: they may have known very different people. At the time of writing, there is considerable dissension between various parties as to how best to memorialize Princess Diana. In a front page article titled 'Archbishop urges end to cult of Diana', we read 'The Archbishop of York . . . has launched a scathing attack on the Diana museum opened last week by the princess's brother, Earl Spencer, on his Althorp estate in Northamptonshire: "It's the last thing she would have wanted"' (*Sunday Times*, 5 July 1998). Many a less high profile family has run into similar difficulties.

The rights of the dead

After a psychotherapist's client died, her middle aged daughter wrote, at the suggestion of her own therapist, to find out what kind of therapy the mother had had. Presumably the daughter's therapist thought it important that her client know more about her mother if she were to know more about herself. The first therapist, however, was crystal clear that therapy was 100 per cent confidential and was surprised any therapist would think otherwise. The daughter also found that her mother had cut out and thrown away some parts of her correspondence with the therapist, indicating a very private woman who did not want her daughter reading this material.

This raises the question of what rights bereaved people have to see all or indeed any information about the deceased? One might say that we all have a responsibility not to keep anything that we do not want our survivors to see and, since no one can assume they may not die tomorrow, we should be ever vigilant – rather like making sure we always have clean underwear on in case we get knocked down by a bus. But always keeping the equivalent of clean underwear in our correspondence is not so easy. Even if we do succeed, we cannot prevent survivors digging. The parent who is a private person, choosing to reveal little of him- or herself, is precisely the kind of parent that surviving children may wish to find out more about. And who is to stop them?

If it is morally right to respect the privacy of the newly dead, how far back should such respect go? The makers of the film *Titanic* were taken to task for misrepresenting someone who had died 85 years earlier. Should we take Shakespeare to task for elaborating, on the basis of very little evidence, characters who had died centuries before? Is it ethical for biographers, refused material by the subject of the biography while still alive, to trawl through hitherto denied correspondence once the subject has died? It can be a tortuous business balancing the desire of the living to copyright the stories that will be told after their demise, the need of some bereaved people to know the truth and the rather different agendas of those who publish history, biography and literature for profit and for posterity. Once again, we see that telling the story of the dead leads into the writing of history.

Summary

The dead live on not only in private memory and experience, but also in conversation among the living. In the absence of ancestor cults and formal religious rites of remembrance, everyday conversation is probably the primary means by which the dead live on in modern society. The chapter began with a number of theoretical perspectives on this, concentrating on Berger's and Giddens's theories about the instability of personal identity in the modern world and the fragmentation of the individual's life experience, notably in the separation of home and work. This means that there is often much about the deceased of which we are ignorant, yet those who know about these other aspects are not readily available to talk to. Fitting together a picture of the dead, and by implication of oneself, is therefore made necessary yet impeded by modern conditions.

The chapter proceeded to look at how this works out in two particular forms of bereavement – widowhood, where the widow has lost her main conversation partner; and student, or similar, bereavements when the mourner is away from home for long periods. Some practical implications are sketched: where family members are unable or unwilling to talk about the dead, the funeral, memory books, mutual help groups and counselling can all provide arenas in which the deceased's story can be told and edited. Finally, two ethical questions are raised: need the story be true? and what rights do the dead themselves have to control their own obituary?

Further reading

Harvey, J. (1996) *Embracing their Memory: Loss and the Social Psychology of Storytelling*. Needham Heights, MA: Allyn & Bacon.

Klass, D. (1997) The deceased child in the psychic and social worlds of bereaved parents during the resolution of grief. *Death Studies*, 21(2): 147–75. (Reprinted in Klass *et al.* (1996) *Continuing Bonds*.)

Walter, T. (1996) A new model of grief: bereavement and biography. *Mortality*, 1(1): 7–25.

Questions

1 In your experience, have you found that people are unwilling to talk about the dead? If so, why is this?
2 Is it your experience that fellow mourners no longer live with one another? What consequences flow from this?
3 Some clients may value counselling because it allows them to talk about the dead person. Do you agree? If so, would this modify your own style of counselling?

Notes

1 In Catholic funerals, a personal tribute may be given by a relative or friend rather than by the priest.
2 Of course the *prime* purpose of a funeral and of counselling are different: in the case of the funeral to pay respect to the dead, in the case of counselling to mitigate the suffering of the bereaved.

5 | The last chapter

For many bereaved people, the single most important part of the story is how and why the person died. This can be a major concern in unexpected and sudden death, and almost always in suicide. A correspondent from the USA wrote to me:

> Recently, I spoke to a man whose 38-year-old son committed suicide. The father made numerous phone calls to his other children, to friends and neighbours and to local shop keepers, obtained newspaper cuttings and police reports and the coroner's report. In this way, he was able to compose a picture of his son's final hours.

Without some sense being made of the death, how can this man make sense of his son's life? All human beings seem to need theodicies, explanations for suffering, without which death throws our world into meaninglessness and anomie (Berger 1969; Nadeau 1998; Neimeyer 1999). Even when a death is expected, the survivor may go over and over it. When Kate Bennett (1998) interviewed widows, she found they talked about the actual death in elaborate narratives, in contrast to the rest of the interview where their contributions were much shorter; these death narratives seem to have been frequently rehearsed, perhaps in order to fix the events in the widow's mind. Littlewood (1992: 46) similarly writes of widows' 'obsessive reviewing of the events that led up to the death'. Even if death is expected, its actual shape and timing may come as a surprise. A close friend died in a hospice of breast cancer, but few of us expected her actual death to be as sudden and painful as it turned out to be and we needed time afterwards with the doctor to go through, in detail, exactly what had happened.

Religious, medical and psychological languages

The language in which last chapters have been written has changed mark-edly over the past four centuries.[1] The account we sought of my friend's death is not the account we would have sought had we lived in the seventeenth century.

From the late Middle Ages onwards, Catholicism emphasized the importance of deathbed behaviour – last minute repentance for major sins, or conversely deathbed apostasy after an exemplary life, could at the very last minute change the course of one's eternal destiny. Although the Reformation was supposed to shift attention from the last hours to the whole of life, the sixteenth and seventeenth centuries in England witnessed even greater interest in the spiritual performance of the dying man or woman (Houlbrooke 1998). Lethargy, delirium, excruciating pain and sudden death rendered many incapable of anything resembling a model deathbed performance, and the more hard line Puritans saw a poor performance as reflecting the person's spiritual, rather than bodily, state. Published accounts of the deathbed performance were often published post-mortem in order finally to define the person, and typically described exemplary forbearing and faith, serving to mark the deceased as one of the elect. Women's deaths could be of special interest. Rehearsed in pain through childbirth (which, of course, was prepared for as a possible death as well as a possible birth), and forbidden to speak in church, their deathbed prayers, exhortations and affirmations of faith were heard with special respect. For someone to be remembered well, it was important that their last words and actions be recorded as those of faith, and doubtless this provided comfort to their survivors that those they loved were now in a better place. The last minute conversions of notorious criminals were of particular interest to the public at large.

Even as late as the nineteenth century, and even among atheists, the last chapter was written in the language of faith. Although secularists claimed that only Christians think it really matters how you die, in practice great interest was shown in the deaths of avowed atheists. It was very important that they did not, at the last moment, recant. Recantation would invalidate their life, just as last minute apostasy would for a Christian (Nash 1996). The last chapter either sums up, or invalidates, the rest of a person's life.

That said, from the eighteenth century the religious interest in the last chapter was undermined as medicine came to augment religion at the deathbed. People were as concerned that a doctor be present capable of administering opium to kill the pain as a priest capable of eliciting faith (Porter 1989). By the twentieth century, we are now more likely to ask 'Did she die in any pain?' or 'What finally killed her?' rather than 'Did she die believing?' In a society that values medical over other accounts of suffering (Frank 1995: ch.1), we turn to the doctor to write the last chapter. Even children now want the medical facts. Winston's Wish, a charity in Gloucestershire for bereaved children, arranges weekends for them, and around the camp-fire the children write questions for the invited doctor to answer. Not so many ask about the emotional aspects of bereavement; many more want to know the physical details of what happens when you die (Thompson 1995). Their interest seems to be both general and specific; they want to know what happens to dead people in general and they want to know what happened to their mummy or daddy. They get the doctor to tell them the last chapter.

Organ transplants now mean that the last part of the person's medical story may be post- rather than pre-mortem. Friends and relatives may find some meaning in the tragically sudden death of a young person if parts of the body have been used to give life to someone else; there may even be visions of the person being, partially, alive in someone else. Sque and Payne (1996) found that relatives wanted information about the recipient, so they could answer the question 'Where is he now?' and write the final bit of the last chapter.

Largely as a result of the influential work of Kübler-Ross (1970, 1975), we may now detect a third shift, from a religious to a medical to a psycho-logical/personal growth version of the last chapter. Kübler-Ross emphas-ized the importance, for both the dying person and their significant others, of completing 'unfinished business', things in their relationships that need sorting out. Once the person has died, the business can never be finished, so having completed things can be as, if not more, important to the survivors than to the dying. Business that was unfinished at the time of death can torment survivors. So the question now may be not so much 'Did he make his peace with his maker before he died?' or even 'Did he die without pain?' but 'Did he make his peace with his father/wife/daughter/son before he died?' The contemporary hospice version of the good death typically entails a social-psychological finishing of the person's business as well as pain management; indeed helping patients to finish psychological business they would rather not face up to may constitute the majority of the staff's labours in certain cases. Unfinished business, or what Saunders (1988) somewhat misleadingly calls spiritual pain, can be at the root of physical pain so that both have to be treated holistically.[2] The last chapters that are published out of the hospice movement (e.g. de Hennezel 1997) may be seen as the personal growth equivalent of the Puritan deathbed account, each making a definitive statement of the character of the person's death and therefore of his or her life, each made in the language of the time, and each comforting those left behind.

This kind of extended last chapter, focusing on personal and interper-sonal growth, is made possible by the long time that cancer or AIDS takes to kill – and is much less likely with diseases such as heart disease whose course is less predictable, or with strokes and Alzheimer's where communica-tion is impaired. Exley (1998) found that cancer patients in a hospice she studied were concerned to make life as easy as possible for their loved ones and actively participated in constructing the memories they would leave behind. The deceased can therefore be co-author, with the bereaved, of the last chapter.

When the last chapter is too painful

Sometimes, with the best will in the world, the last chapter may make grim reading. In a North American study of adolescent sibling bereavement, 36 per cent of those interviewed expressed blame, guilt or shame about what they felt was their inability to help their dying sibling or to prevent the death. This usually followed suicide, homicide or accidental death:

> It was harder for me to cope with my brother's death mainly because I was the one who found him after his suicide. He had hung himself, and I had to get him down by myself and go get help. The picture of him hanging there is always on my mind, and I can never forget it. Also, my mom kept badgering me to go get him for supper, and I kept saying 'wait a minute'. The life-saving crew said that if I had come down two minutes sooner and got him down his brain would have had enough oxygen, and he would have lived. But because of my stubbornness to do work, he died.

> Seeing how much guilt I have inside me. I was gone all day and didn't get home until around 9.00 that night, and he was sick; but we thought it was just flu. He started making weird breathing sounds, like he couldn't breathe. I started yelling at him to stop faking. It was only 10 minutes later that he collapsed and died right there.
>
> (Hogan and DeSantis 1994: 139)

Such people wish utterly to erase the last chapter, but cannot. Their stories warn us against the romantic idea that writing the final chapter will necessarily comfort. They might be able slightly to rewrite the story in order to lessen their guilt – maybe nobody would have recognized it wasn't flu, it's not a sin to be conscientious over one's homework – but ultimately the facts cannot be changed. With the best will in the world, some people are implicated in – or at least have witnessed – the ghastly deaths of those they love.

Often, no relative has witnessed such deaths, but various officials – doctors, nurses, ambulance or police crew, fellow soldiers – have. The relatives want to know what happened. How much of the truth should those who know actually tell? Some officials may have their own reasons for hiding the truth, for fear of litigation, and how do bureaucratically or legally required investigations into the cause of death mesh, or not mesh, with relatives' need for an account of what happened? It is with these deaths that 'writing the last chapter' can become a major concern for doctors, nurses, police officers, coroners, insurance companies and soldiers as well as for relatives, and can become a major source of tension between the parties.[3]

A death at the front

Dying in war away from home has been all too common a lot for twentieth-century men. How do kin back home write the last chapter? In World War One, as in subsequent wars, officers wrote official and stylized letters to inform next of kin of the circumstances in which their young man died, while the Red Cross followed up thousands of cases in order to find more information (Winter 1995: 35–44). The accounts that flowed home were typically of heroic death, in many cases covering up truly unspeakable circumstances. Other comrades would take it upon themselves to provide further information.

The section that follows consists of letters that document my grand-mother's experience of (literally) writing the last chapter of her eldest son, my father's older brother, Argyll. The letters are reproduced in full, in order to reveal the concerns of their authors. Arg's death at the front on 9 May 1915 was recorded in the local London paper, *The Hornsey Journal* on 28 May, and shortly afterwards my grandmother received the following unsolicited letter:

> Pte R.S. Eason (no.2345)
> 13th (Kensington) Battln.
> London Reg.
> Cavalry Corps Railhead
> June 1st '15

Dear Mrs Walters,
A few lines to let you know that my mother has written asking me if I could find out anything of how your son died. One of my friends who was with him till the last told me he lost his life doing a brave deed.

As you know on that Sunday morning we were ordered to take 3 lines of trenches from the Germans. This we did, your son succeeding in getting into the third German trench having to cross an open piece of ground which was swept by rifle fire.

When they had got into the trench it was found that a flag, which was used to mark our position, had been left behind. As it was essen-tial that we should have the flag the officer in command asked for

volunteers to go and fetch it. Almost before he had finished your son
was out of the trench running as hard as he could and was within five
yards of it when he fell. He was not seen to move again. The time this
happened was just about 10 o'c Sunday morning, a day I shall never
forget.

    I must close now + trust that this will be a comfort to you to know
your son died a noble death.

        I am Yours sincerely
           R.S. Eason

The writer constructs the death as heroic, indicating a level of bravery that
might have deserved posthumous decoration, but certainly intended to comfort my grandmother. This was soon followed by another unsolicited letter
from a soldier who knew nothing about the actual death, but knew the
desire of mothers to know how their sons died and so took it upon himself
to write his own idealized version of Arg's last hours in the belief that it
would comfort my grandmother. He believed that general information about
the offensive would help her, even though he could tell her nothing specifically about her son.

June 1915

Dear Mrs Walter.

You will be very surprised to hear from me + the only introduction
I offer is that I happen to live in Crouch End + am now serving with
the 7th Middlesex Regt at the Front. I have just received from home
a copy of the Hornsey Journal in which I regret to notice the an-
nouncement of your great bereavement and that you are unaware of
the circumstances of your brave son's death.

    Although I am sorry I cannot give you any actual details of how he
fell – I, as one who took part in the same action – happened to witness
the glorious charge of the 'Kensingtons' on that date. The battle was
fought in the district of Fromelles on the morning of May 9th. At
4 a.m. a terrific artillery bombardment commenced which lasted for
the greater part of an hour – a few minutes before 5 o'clock, 125 yards
of German trench was blown up by one of our mines – and this was
the signal for the 'Kensingtons' to charge. I shall never forget that
sight! they were actually the first battalion over the parapet + the way
they fought through three lines of German trenches will stand, I am
sure, as one of the most gallant feats of this great war. I notice that you
mention he was a 'bomber' + I am pleased to tell you that the bombers
did magnificent work on that day.

    Well, Madam, I hope you will excuse me for writing you on this
occasion but I am pleased to be able to let one poor Mother know that

her son died as 'a gallant Kensington' bomber in that glorious charge at Fromelles.

> I am, Madam,
> Yours very sincerely,
> Albert E. Ascott

PS At present I am some considerable distance from this battlefield but if I ever I have an opportunity of finding the grave of your poor son, I shall let you know immediately through Mr. J.G. Steele of Park Road, with whom I am constantly in touch.

More remarkable is a letter received after the end of the war from a German soldier.

> Bad Aibling
> 19th October 1919

I allow myself to send you a letter which was found on an English soldier who fell near Fromelles, North France, on 9th May 1915.

The letter was addressed to Mr. H. Walter, London and River Plate Bank Ltd, Rio de Janeiro, Brazil.

He fell in my neighbourhood and I think he is a near relative of yours; therefore I am sending you this letter.

He fell on 9th May 1915, when storming our positions – a brave soldier fighting for his Country.

It is my business to deal with the correspondence of opponents and that is why I took this letter. I have no knowledge whatever as to the remainder of his effects.

If you desire any further information – as to the fight, the manner of his death, and of his grave, I am at your service.

> Peter Ehrhardt
> Police Sergeant
> Bad Aibling, Bayern, Germany

It seems that my grandmother indeed requested further information, receiving the following reply:

> Bad Aibling Nov 20th '19

Mrs E.A. Walter, London

Acknowledging receipt of your favor of the 12th inst. I hasten to give you herewith, as far as I remember particulars of the death of your respected son.

On the 15th of April '15 I came to an Infantry Regiment belonging to the 6th Bavarian Reserve Division + which was stationed near Fromelles (on the left from Ill and directly south of Armentieres). Here at the beginning it was fairly quiet until the 9th of May when about half past four in the morning heavy English Artillery fire started.

We laid under cover for an hour on account of heavy drum-firing when suddenly with a terrible explosion of the 3rd shot of our Company we were blown into the air and, as was found out later, the next Company to our left was also blown up having been undermined by the English.

Through the breach thus made in our line came forward an English regiment which attacked us part from the front, part from the back.

Your respected son who, as a grenade thrower, must have come on amongst the first, started throwing hand-grenades into our position.

We found ourselves in a very queer situation and defended ourselves for our lives.

Your respected son fell on the named date about 6 a.m. through a rifle shot and several hand grenade splinters and was killed on the spot.

From the English Regiment which carried out their duty so valiantly very few remained alive (of about 3000 men, between 2400 + 2500 were killed).

But we too had very heavy losses as, through the explosion alone my Company lost 92 men.

The dead were, during the next few days, carried away and interred together in trench-graves on the North West end of the shell-destroyed village of Fromelles; military honors, as we were in the habit of rendering, could here not be rendered, as the work could only be carried out at night when we were often subjected to English machine-gun and artillery fire.

The trench-graves of the fallen comrades near Fromelles would not, very likely, look so nice as would be wished for the brave comrades buried there as, in the course of time, and through the numerous battles subsequently fought in that part, they would be no doubt often disturbed.

Your respected son had, no doubt, several more letters on him but, as mentioned before, I took interest only in the one from a near relative; other things like his purse, ring, etc, I would not take nor did I allow them to be taken by anyone else near by as it would be a heavy responsibility to take any valuables away. Either from friend or foe.

Your fallen son had two addressed covers [envelopes] with him, the one which I deemed to be to your dear address and one addressed to an uncle of his in America.

Though I should willingly do so, if it were at all possible for me, I am sorry I cannot tell you what became of the other belongings of your cherished son.

I am awfully sorry not to be able to give your daughter any information about the missing Mr. H.J. Savage, as it is likely the poor man must have fallen at our offensive on the Kemmel Ridge where both sides lost so heavily.

It would please me greatly if I could bring you some peace of mind with the above particulars as it is too hard for a poor mother to know only so little of her dear ones.

Underneath I thought of drawing a little sketch of the neighbourhood for your information.

Will you kindly acknowledge receipt of this letter and from time to time let me hear from you.

    Kindly share with your family
        the numerous friendly respects
        from
           Yours truly
           Peter Ehrhardt
           Police Sergeant

Seven decades later, I, being Arg's nephew, took an interest in the matter and received the following information about his place of burial, which, I guess, really is the final chapter. The story of a person's life cannot be finally told until it is known if, and where, they are buried.

Commonwealth War Graves Commission
2 Marlow Road
Maidenhead
Berkshire
5 March 1991

Dear Mr Walter
Thank you for your recent letter. I confirm the following information from our records.

Private Argyle Francis Bradford Walter, 2795, serving with 13th Kensington Battalion, London Regiment, died on 9 May 1915, age 22 and, sadly, has no known grave. His name, along with others from his Regiment, appears on Panels 10 and 11 of the Ploegsteert Memorial, Belgium. He was the son of Ellen Annie Walter of Muswell Hill, London, and the late Francis Edward Walter.

The village of Ploegsteert is about 16 kilometres south of Ieper (formerly Ypres), near the Franco-Belgian border and about 5 kilometres north of Armentieres. The Ploegsteert Memorial stands in Berks

Cemetery Extension, about 2 kilometres north of the village on the west side of the road to Ieper.

I hope you will find this information helpful.

All these versions of how he died are fairly consistent, though idealized and certainly the horror of war is not in them. He may have lain for hours in agony. The last chapter we have of Arg's life is probably accurate, but very far from complete. My grandmother received no religious, medical or psychological details of her son's last moments, but the military facts were the discourse of the day and out of them an account of heroism was constructed for her. She was lucky: she was told a story, it was a good story, it received independent and unsolicited confirmation, and it seems to have been believed. Whether my aunt, aged 18 at the end of the war, ever found out what happened to her friend Mr. H.J. Savage, I do not know. Many soldiers have no known grave, others were reported missing in action, presumed dead, with no further information available.

Others are killed by 'friendly fire', which the official account may do its best to cover up; the family may or may not suspect the truth. In World War Two, hundreds of American GIs killed in exercises in preparation for D-Day were reported to families back home as 'missing in action' – even though the military had recovered, identified and buried the bodies – in order to maintain secrecy about the planned invasion of France, but this secrecy was maintained for decades after it was strategically necessary. British as well as American commanders, embarrassed by a fiasco that turned to tragedy, left relatives wondering whether their man might perhaps be a prisoner-of-war and might one day return. The powerful covering their backsides usually wins over the needs of mourners to know at least something of the truth (Small 1989). Blank (1998: 165) claims that the American military still reveal no more than they want to about deaths in service, which can be very little indeed.

The soldier and his family may have very different evaluations of the war. Käthe Kollwitz struggled with the knowledge that her understanding of the last chapter of her young son's life was at odds with his own understanding, a struggle that inspired her moving sculpture in the cemetery in Flanders where her son is buried. He died in October 1914 in the first flush of optimism about the war.

'Is it a break of faith with you, Peter', she wrote in October 1916, 'if I can now see only madness in the war?' He had died believing; how could his mother not honour that belief? But to feel that the war was an exercise in futility led to the even more damaging admission that her son and his whole generation had been 'betrayed'. This recognition was agonizing, but she did not flinch from giving it artistic form. This is one reason why it took so long for her to complete the monument, and why she and her husband are on their knees before their son's grave. They are there to beg his forgiveness, to ask him to accept their failure to find a better way, their failure to prevent the madness of war from cutting his life short.

(Winter 1995: 110–1)

How many Americans have echoed these words after Vietnam?

I have yet to visit Arg's memorial, or the battlefield on which he fell, but many soldiers' relatives and descendants have. For them, there seem to be at least two components to their pilgrimage. First, visiting the grave, seeing the name carved in stone, can be an emotional experience, substituting for the funeral they never attended. Second, walking the ground on which the man fell, along with talking to tour leaders and old soldiers, enables a picture to be drawn of what might have happened and is more a cognitive experience. Both may be necessary for some to lay their dead finally to rest (Walter 1993c).

Accidental death and unlawful killing

At the Hillsborough soccer stadium disaster in 1989, Liverpool fans were crowded into one end of the ground and 94 were crushed to death in full view of both police security cameras and live national television cameras covering the match. Press use of close-up photographs of the dead and dying caused distress for many people, but photographs and especially video material were later used to help both survivors of the crush and bereaved relatives to work out exactly where they, or their loved ones, had been standing, what had happened and why. Newburn (1993: 111, 119) found that those who received social work intervention after the disaster found it helpful to be able to talk about what happened, over and over again in painfully explicit detail. This enabled them both to validate their feelings and to piece together what happened – the equivalent of re-visiting the battlefield in order to work out exactly what had happened.

If understanding what happened at Hillsborough was important for many, understanding why it happened was even more important for some. Certain sections of the press implied that Liverpool fans, widely vilified as hooligans, had brought the crush upon themselves by their unruly behaviour. No evidence whatsoever for this was found, but it is still believed in some quarters, especially abroad where the death of any English soccer fan is assumed to be self-inflicted. There was, however, considerable evidence for the disaster having been caused by police incompetence and callousness toward fans, so families were dismayed when the coroner gave a verdict not of unlawful killing but of accidental death. A police officer who committed perjury at the coroner's court by giving the false impression that none of the dead suffered was believed by some families to be trying to protect the police rather than the feelings of the bereaved.[4]

The handling by coroner's courts of road traffic accidents can lead to similar kinds of distress (Howarth 1997). Of the 4500 road deaths in the UK in 1991, only 416 resulted in prosecution, the rest going no further than the coroner's court, whose remit is not to establish blame but simply to establish who died, when and of what physical cause. Friends and relatives, by contrast, often want the coroner to establish blame and feel cheated when the verdict simply states the medical details and concludes that the person died accidentally. Howarth found that others go to the inquest because they want to hear exactly what happened – most kin were not at the scene of the accident, are not able to read official reports and may have found eye witnesses unwilling to tell them the details:

I wanted to go to the inquest because I wanted to know what had happened and I couldn't get anyone to tell me. I think they were protecting me. People don't seem to realise that you need to know.

Sitting through the inquest was awful; listening to the accounts of what happened and hearing the pathologist's report. But at least I now know how it happened.

(Howarth 1997: 153, 152)

Families want to know what happened in order that they can 'write the last chapter', but the coroner's court exists to satisfy certain legal requirements, not to assuage grief. Some coroners will be sensitive to this, but it is not what they are there for, and they cannot get involved in discussions of blame. What makes it more complicated is that some families may find the coroner's court provides too much information, revealing gory details they would rather be spared. Worse, some of this information may be in excess of what is required to establish the facts of the case, and is experienced by the family as gratuitous (Biddle 1998). This is because the court's discourse is legal–medical, and coroner and witnesses have to choose to step out of this frame to consider the personal feelings of any family present.

All accidental deaths have to be investigated by the police so that they can assure themselves that they are not in fact dealing with a case of cleverly concealed murder or suicide. This frequently causes distress to the next of kin. Parents already in shock at finding their previously healthy baby dead in its cot find themselves within hours being questioned by a police officer who needs to ascertain that this was in truth a cot death rather than infanticide. Within hours of their daughter falling off an open-platform London bus and being run over, Pamela Elder and her husband faced police officers trying to ascertain whether this might have been suicide rather than a freak accident. The parents were seeking the facts of what happened, but left the police station 'deeply disturbed and angry at the total lack of sensitivity' (Elder 1998: 119).

A mutual help organization for bereaved parents comments on murder and road deaths:

> The lack of awareness and of sensitivity shown by 'authority' . . . leaves many parents and other relatives with the feeling that the victim's life was of no value, of no significance to society. Where death occurs in an employment situation, similar feelings can arise. All these are exacerbated by insurance companies refusing to allow their clients to express regret and sorrow, lest this be taken as an admission of guilt and therefore liability.
>
> (Compassionate Friends Spring Newsletter 1992: 16)

The body – often in a bad state – has to be identified, which may or may not fit with the family's desire or lack of desire to see it. This final chapter of a person's life is typically an illustrated chapter, vividly illuminated by the final sighting of the corpse.

Such deaths dramatize the conflict, identified by Prior (1989) and Walter (1994), between the public responsibilities of medicine, the law and bureaucracy and the private needs of dying and bereaved individuals. The hospice movement and other holistic approaches have tried to bring the two together, with considerable success in the case of slow cancer deaths, but where deaths are sudden or potentially unlawful then legal requirements lead to a fragmented experience for bereaved families. The police and other authorities are in a no-win situation: the requirements of the law and the needs of the bereaved are in some senses incompatible. At worst, maybe all that can be achieved is greater sensitivity in an impossible situation; the UK has seen a number of articles recently in the police press attempting to foster better practice in this area (Cathcart and Kerr 1996; Dix 1997; Harrison 1998). At best, it may be possible, as I discuss in a later section on Scotland, that the legal requirement to gather information and the humanitarian drive to provide relatives with information could be married more effectively.

Murder brings the bereaved and society into very specific tensions (Riches and Dawson 1998). Whether through media reporting or gossip, the identity of the deceased and by extension the family may be 'spoiled' (Goffman 1963). Murder in the violent world of drugs or petty crime suggests that the victim as well as the perpetrator was involved in this world, and implies that the victim's parents had done a less than good job in raising him or her. After the murder of a child outside of the home, others may wonder if the parents should have been more vigilant in keeping an eye on their toddler or more knowledgeable about where their teenage daughter was at that hour. After murder by a stranger (Rock 1998), the survivor's (e.g. parent's or spouse's) image of an orderly universe is shattered. The entire life of both victim and survivor is re-written in the light of this unexpected and dominating event, separating survivors from those friends and relatives with whom they had once had so much in common, but now share nothing.

The court can also spoil the victim's identity. A mother writes about her 15-year-old, killed by her ex-boyfriend on her way home from shopping: 'The victim obviously cannot be present at the trial, therefore someone should be able to voice the character of the victim, not to leave the defence to paint a false, and in their own interest, character of the victim.' She goes on to say that reducing the sentence from murder to manslaughter reduced the value of her daughter's life (Compassionate Friends Spring 1992 Newsletter, p.17; see also Rock 1998). Relatives of those who died in the December 1988 explosion of PanAm flight 103 over the Scottish town of Lockerbie were, a decade later, upset because the Libyan government had still not released the two men suspected of the bombing, claiming that they would not get a fair trial in Scotland. The British government did not wish to lose face by acceding to Libyan demands to hold the trial elsewhere. Politico-legal wrangling was thus delaying indefinitely the production of an officially certified account of the deaths (*The Times* 27 October 1997).

In the months and sometimes years after a disaster, the media return periodically to the story, when an interim official report is published, when the final report is published, when the trial (if there is one) begins, when the verdict is made, and so on. These reminders of the death arrive in the home of bereaved families via the television screen, often unexpected. Getting through grief at their own chosen pace is interrupted, and they have to move at the erratic pace of the media and of officialdom. Each time, there may be a new twist to the story, which causes revision of the final chapter. The press as much as officialdom can be the origin of these stories. At the time of writing, nine months after her death, every week or so a newspaper produces a new claim as to Princess Diana's last moments. 'Gendarme tells of Diana's last words . . . The last thing Princess Diana saw before she died was the body of Dodi Fayed lying next to her, it was claimed today' (*Evening Standard* 25 June 1998). It seems unlikely that her two sons would welcome this constant revision of the gory last chapter of their mother's life.

In some states in the USA, the victim's family can choose to watch the convicted murderer's execution.[5] Witnessing this really final episode may not be approved of by all, but given what families will have had to go through on the way, one can see why some take up this option not to be excluded at the very end of a legal process that has continued for years with scant regard for their feelings. In previous centuries, of course, hangings were public and attracted large crowds, and it is only in the contemporary West that executions have become as a matter of course private. How this interacts with the desire of bereaved families to write the last chapter is unknown.

In Chapter 2, I mentioned communal remembering by groups of combatants. Similar groups can form following mass disasters in which a number of people suffer the same unusual bereavement. Following the burial of the Aberfan primary school in 1966 (Miller 1974), the Lockerbie air crash, the Hillsborough disaster, the Dunblane school shooting and other unique disasters, bereaved families bonded together into mutual help groups that provided emotional support and some of which also fought for justice. To be bereaved sets you apart from everyone else, and to be bereaved in such unusual circumstances sets you apart even more; but unlike most bereavements you are in the company of others who have suffered the same trauma, will face the same challenges and will suffer again on the same anniversaries. Such people can form intense bonds. They share each others' stories and (as with Hillsborough) may together construct their communal version of what happened, over against the official version.

Implications

Relatives often want to know more about how the person died. This can put those in the know – whether doctors, emergency personnel, or fellow soldiers – in a difficult position. Sudnow's (1967: 146) classic study of how medical staff routinely handle death showed how, in the Californian hospitals he studied, both the breaking of the initial news and the further information was routinely handled in a way designed to minimize distress to the family (and thus to minimize disruption in the ward). A study of British pathologists found much the same

> I know we can't say with any great accuracy . . . but we usually come out and tell them, you know, probably they wouldn't have *suffered* . . . Everything had happened so quickly. You know . . . we don't know: we weren't there. The chap could have been holding onto his chest for ever for all we know, and all they know. But they're usually quite happy. And then they go away quite satisfied, thinking 'it was all very quick.' . . . And they can go back an' get on with their own post-mortem, if you like.
>
> (Silverman and Bloor 1990: 9)

Reports home from war fronts are doubtless similarly tailored. Seale (1998) argues that such accounts not only 'inform' the relative about the nature of the death, but also help to restore an orderly world, a world in which people die swiftly, whether of heart attacks or enemy bullets, a world in which cancer pain is controlled.

With increasing education of patients, and increasing informality between patients and doctors (Wouters 1990), the numbers of families who ask doctors to tell them the details of the patient's final hours are probably increasing. Such families will be less and less easily fobbed off with half truths, and medical units are now having to take this aspect of bereavement care more seriously. First palliative care units, and now accident and emergency units (Royal College of Nursing 1995) and other specialties, are considering bereavement care. Key questions are: to what extent should this be conducted by a specialist bereavement unit rather than by medical and nursing staff themselves going over the details of the death? Is counselling – the construction and editing of a story about the death – best done by staff who knew the patient or by a specialist counsellor who never met the deceased? Home care cancer nurses often pop in to see their families several times after the death, even though this may not be part of their job description. To what extent do they, as well as the families, need to go over the story as part of their own grieving?

Some accident and emergency units are now giving relatives the choice to witness resuscitation attempts and a recent pilot study at Addenbrooke's Hospital, Cambridge (Robinson *et al.* 1998) found that witnessing a failed resuscitation attempt did not add to the trauma of loss; indeed staff became convinced of its positive benefit. The study's authors speculate this may be because it builds up a relation between staff and relatives before staff have to break the bad news, but another (not incompatible) possibility is that it provides greater certainty in writing the last chapter.

A second area of concern in the UK are post-mortem procedures. Around 150,000 autopsies are carried out each year, that is, on more than one corpse in four, although only 1500 cases involve any suspicion of crime. The remainder are carried out for medical reasons, to ascertain the cause of death, to learn if the diagnosis was correct, and to learn about life-threatening complications following treatment. Autopsies often reveal that the actual cause of death is other than that suspected, throwing doubt on the accuracy of 75 per cent of death certificates. Such are the medical arguments for such a large number of autopsies (Knight 1997), but questions are being asked about the effects on bereaved people and whether too many post-mortems are conducted (Scotland, for example, has proportionately half as many as England and Wales). The corpse is the property of the state during this period, and the medical–legal process takes little account of the family. A system devised out of nineteenth-century medical concerns is being challenged at the end of the twentieth century by those more concerned with the psychological health of the bereaved. Busuttil (1998) emphasizes the importance of good communication between pathologist and the bereaved.

Third, and related to post-mortems, are coroner's courts. Some interesting changes are afoot in Scotland where unexpected deaths are investigated not in public by the coroner, but in private by the procurator fiscal, who also makes the decision whether or not to start a prosecution. In the wake of Scottish disasters such as the Lockerbie bombing, the fire on the Piper Alpha oil platform and the shooting of sixteen 5-year-old schoolchildren at Dunblane, fiscals increasingly see a significant part of their job as the regular giving of information to relatives, which may be done over a period of time as the fiscal's private investigations proceed. After the Dunblane shooting, the fiscal regularly and promptly passed information onto the families so that they did not need to learn anything second-hand from the press (Ruxton and Miller 1998).

Fourth, the culture of suing, largely North American but increasing in the UK, means that officials are reluctant to tell the truth to bereaved families, for fear of opening themselves or their organizations to a financial claim. The more families in general sue, the less any one family can expect to get the information necessary to write the last chapter. A family's desire to blame and to get compensation militates against the desire simply to know what happened. This raises the question of whether the kind of amnesty pioneered (in a very specific historical situation) by South Africa's Truth and Reconciliation Commission might somehow be applied to more everyday deaths in other countries. Without such a development, the desire of medics and officials to cover their backsides and the desire of families to know what happened will become ever more incompatible.

Palliative care has succeeded in demonstrating new ways of bringing institutional arrangements more in line with the personal experience of patients and their families, linking public provision and private experience in a new 'postmodern' synthesis (Walter 1994). The reduction of total pain (psychological, social and existential as well as physical) has been a priority. It remains to be seen whether comparable creativity will be manifested in humanizing the legal, medical and bureaucratic routines that follow sudden death, so that they minimize, or at least do not exacerbate, the pain felt by bereaved families.

Summary

The language in which the good, or bad, death is recounted has shifted over time from a religious, to a medical, to a psychological language. The very last chapter of a person's life may be traumatic, with the mourner wishing to erase it from memory; or it may be enigmatic, with the mourner seeking an account of the death from officials present at the time: doctors, nurses, rescue personnel, fellow soldiers. If the death was hard, these officials are likely to be compassionately selective with the truth: deaths at the front are heroic and instant, deaths in hospital are peaceful. Deaths that result in public proceedings in a court of law – following, for example, suicide, murder or disaster – are altogether more problematic and typically entail a conflict between, on the one hand, the interests of justice, the press and other interest groups for certain kinds of accounts, and on the other hand the mourners' needs for an account that minimizes the death's badness. The chapter closes with a discussion of how to reform procedures in hospitals, post-mortems, coroner's courts, and other settings in which deaths have to be publicly accounted for.

Further reading

Howarth, G. (1997) Death on the road: the role of the English coroner's court in the social construction of an accident, in M. Mitchell (ed.) *The Aftermath of Road Accidents*. London: Routledge.

Rock, P. (1998) *After Homicide: Practical and Political Responses to Bereavement*. Oxford: Clarendon Press.

Walter, T. (1996) A new model of grief: bereavement and biography. *Mortality*, 1(1): 7–25.

Wells, C. (1994) Disasters: the role of institutional responses in shaping public perceptions of death, in R. Lee and D. Morgan (eds) *Death Rites: Law and Ethics at the End of Life*. London: Routledge.

Questions

1 The protracted procedures of the law are often incompatible with the needs of the bereaved to know as soon as possible as much of what happened as they can bear and then be left in peace. Are there ways in which the two could be brought more into harmony?

2 What obligation do nurses, doctors, chaplains or other personnel have to tell the truth to the family when the death was a bad one? What rights do the family have to know, or not to know?

3 How might the routines of medical or para-medical facilities be restructured to accommodate families who wish to be told about, or even to witness, the last minutes of a person's life?

Notes

1 I take the term 'last chapter' from the gerontologist Victor Marshall (1986), modifying it in the process. Marshall's last chapter, the reminiscence or life review (Butler 1963) conducted by the old person, I see as the penultimate chapter. The last chapter, I suggest, is written after the person's death, by others – at the funeral, in obituaries and in conversation. Of course, an old person's own review of his or her life may entail writing the last chapters of deceased friends and family members.

2 I say misleadingly, because it has much more to do with existential notions of meaning and with contemporary psychological notions of personal growth than with traditional concepts of the spiritual, which in the West typically have entailed

some notion of God and an afterlife. 'Existential pain', Malcolm Johnson's term 'biographical pain', or Saunders's term 'total pain' would be more appropriate.

3 I do not look at the situation where the body is never found, and where only guesses can be made as to what happened. In peacetime, let alone in war, a surprising number of people simply disappear without trace.

4 *Hillsborough*. ITV, 5 December 1996.

5 Hugo Bedau, personal communication.

6 Theories

The twentieth century has spawned a number of theories of grief – for introductory overviews from various perspectives, see Silverman and Klass (1996), Stroebe and Stroebe (1987), Fraley and Shaver (forthcoming) and Parkes (forthcoming). In this chapter I ask what theoreticians and clinicians have said about continuing bonds between the living and the dead, whether there is currently a revolution going on in thinking about this, and if so what might have caused the revolution.

First, a thumbnail sketch of the theoretical field. Parkes (1998b) distinguishes between *models*, which describe and categorize observed phenomena, and *theories*, which attempt to explain and to find causes. Although this distinction may not be as clear as Parkes suggests, he has usefully delineated the major forms of scientific thinking about grief. He identifies three influential models: (1) the phase model that attempts to classify the processes of grieving; (2) the medical model that notes that grief has many similarities with sickness; and (3) the grief work model that documents the painful effort that is required to make real the fact of loss. All have received considerable criticism.

Parkes identifies four traditional theories of grief: (1) The stress and crisis theory explains grief reactions in terms of the responses to stress that humans have evolved over millennia (Stroebe and Stroebe 1987: ch.5). (2) In Freudian and psychoanalytic theories, mental pain is typically repressed, so bringing the repressed material to consciousness may be required in order to relieve psychiatric symptoms (Freud 1917/1984; Lindemann 1944). This links neatly with the grief work model. (3) The attachment theory was developed by the psychoanalyst, John Bowlby, from his research on children separated from their parents; Bowlby (1961, 1969–1980) and Parkes (1972) later applied attachment theory to bereavement through death. Given the long period that young humans are dependent on their parents, attachment behaviour must have evolved as necessary to survival and is now deeply rooted in the human constitution. (4) The psycho-social transition theory (Marris 1974; Parkes 1993) explains bereavement behaviour in terms of the need to adopt new roles, skills and identities and to review one's world-view.

Theories and bonds

Do the models acknowledge and the theories explain continuing bonds between the living and the dead, and if so how convincing are their explanations? At first sight, the answers to these questions seem to be no. By far the most influential early publication on grief was Freud's article 'Mourning and Melancholia', published in 1917, just as the Victorian celebration of the bond between living and dead was giving way to a twentieth century that found this morbid, that preferred a more muted, more private grief and that found it hard to incorporate the dead into the ongoing life of increasingly secular families and societies. In this context, Freud famously wrote:

> Reality-testing has shown that the loved object no longer exists, and it proceeds to demand that all libido shall be withdrawn from its attachments to that object. This demand arouses understandable opposition ... people never willingly abandon a libidinal position ... Normally, respect for reality gains the day. Nevertheless its orders cannot be obeyed at once. They are carried out bit by bit, at great expense of time and cathectic energy, and in the meantime the existence of the lost object is psychically prolonged ... The fact is, however, that when the work of mourning is completed the ego becomes free and uninhibited again.
>
> (Freud 1917/1984: 253)

We see here many of the ideas that have informed both theory and clinical interventions: ultimately, the dead must be left behind, but this is painful work and so mourners prolong the imagined presence of the dead until, bit by bit, they can accept reality. Attachments to the dead exist, then, but in healthy mourning they are sooner or later left behind. Realism must eventually triumph over romanticism (which could be glossed as the twentieth century must triumph over the nineteenth). The subsequent dominance of this idea that bonds must eventually be broken has been documented by Stroebe *et al.* (1992) and Silverman and Klass (1996) who find it in Bowlby, Parkes, Worden and other leading theorists. In Bowlby and Parkes's attachment theory, for example, searching for a lost object has been adaptive in evolutionary terms: those youngsters who have learnt to search for their parents when temporarily separated are the ones who have survived. In this view, searching is an instinctive response to loss, but one that – in the case of loss through death – will ultimately prove fruitless. It convinces the mourner that the person really will not return and that they must get on with life without them.

Some questions, however, demand further inspection. Were these theorists unaware of the existence of enduring rather than just temporary bonds with the dead? That seems hardly likely, given that only a few decades earlier popular Victorian culture had positively celebrated the immortality of these bonds, producing paintings and poetry still widely circulated today. Or did they, as Silverman and Klass (1996) and Klass (1987–8) suggest, have the data, but ignore and/or misinterpret it? Or did they, as Parkes (1998a) suggests, both have the data and produce intelligent interpretations of it? Or was it, as I have suggested (Walter 1996b), that they did discuss the phenomenon but it was never more than a minor theme in their work and got lost as their theories were passed down via clinicians to the public?

Silverman and Klass seem to be correct for Freud, Volkan, the early Bowlby and a number of other psychoanalysts. Freud certainly did not become 'free and uninhibited again' following the death of his daughter Sophie in her mid-twenties and the death shortly after that of her little boy; he observed that after that he was never able to make any new attachments (Silverman and Klass 1996: 6). Yet Freud never integrated his own experience into his writings on grief.

There are others in the psychoanalytic tradition, however, who have used Freud's concept of internalization to argue that the long-term (and healthy) state of bereaved people is not to leave the dead behind but to incorporate aspects of the person into their own being. In Freudian theory, the child internalizes the parent (the parental voice within), so why should that end just because the parent has died? If aspects of a parent can be internalized, why not aspects of a spouse, child or other significant person? Many in the psychoanalytic tradition write of the internalization of the deceased as something more than a temporary state. Pincus (1976), for example, sensitively identifies different ways in which this can occur in widowhood, depending on the nature of the marital relationship. Parkes (1986: 88) quotes in very positive terms a moving passage from C.S. Lewis (1961) in which, as he begins to let go of his dead wife, Lewis begins to gain a clearer picture of her that he can cherish indefinitely.

Bowlby's early work on young children separated from their mothers identified the children protesting, then despairing and yearning, and eventually protecting themselves by detaching from the mother (to the distress of the mother if and when she returned); it was from this work that he argued that all forms of mourning lead toward detachment (1979: 49). The title of his (1979) book *The Making and Breaking of Affectional Bonds* says it all. Only a year later (1980: 96), however, he observed that 'half or more of widows and widowers reach a state of mind in which they retain a strong sense of the continuing presence of their partner' and this may be necessary if they are to preserve a sense of identity and reorganize their lives. Bowlby knew from this early work that strong attachments are necessary for creative adaptation to change. Bowlby further noted that 'Failure to recognise that a continuing sense of the dead person's presence ... is a common feature of healthy mourning has led to much confused theorising' and he explicitly refuted Freud's view that the function of mourning is 'to detach the survivor's memories and hopes from the dead' (1980: 100).[1]

I will not pursue further the potentially endless debate as to what past theorists did or did not say, and whether they ignored the data or whether they misinterpreted it. The perpetual writing and re-writing of psychoanalytic history can get pretty tedious. The main points I want to make are first that, whatever the theorists did or did not say, a clinical lore developed among bereavement workers that emphasized the breaking of bonds and second that awareness of continuing bonds has increased markedly since the 1980s.[2]

Clinical lore

Klass et al.'s Continuing Bonds (1996) presents a range of research material on the continuing relation to the dead and the sense by many bereaved people that grief never ends; the authors wish to debunk the idea that the function of grief is to sever ties to the dead. In a highly critical review, Parkes (1998a: 28) says that 'The truth is that all of these things have been known for a long time and there are few, if any, people working in the field of bereavement and loss who believe or ever have believed in the myths as stated by the authors.' Parkes is correct that these things have been known about for a long time, but incorrect that hardly any people working in the field had ever believed that the purpose of grief was to sever ties.

In 1996 I published an article (Walter 1996b) in which I argued that the purpose of grief is not to break the bond with the dead but to integrate the dead into the survivor's ongoing life.[3] Hardly a new thesis as far as the scholarly literature was concerned and yet I subsequently received a sizeable mailbag from bereaved people who had somehow or other stumbled across this scholarly article, many of them expressing relief that what they had felt all along had at last been legitimated. These people had received counselling and read umpteen books on bereavement, yet nowhere had they received permission to find a place for their dead. Everywhere the message they had heard was 'Let go. Leave behind. Move on.' One woman wrote:

For over three years I have been grappling with how to move on. My whole instinct has been to construct a 'durable biography' that will enable me to integrate the memory of him into my ongoing life, but you are the first person I have read who has formulated this clearly for me. To this end, I have had an idea to write my son's story, but have so far felt paralysed in this endeavour. (In) all the grief books I have read, nowhere have I found the notion of integrating the dead into my ongoing life.

(From a woman whose son had committed
suicide three years earlier)

Another correspondent wrote:

Eight years after the death of my daughter, health professionals and others consider that I have not 'let go' of her and any health problem I have is attributed to this . . . Why do we concentrate so much on the importance of letting go as a magical formula for recovery?

Another woman, who gave my article to a bereaved colleague, wrote to me that after eight years 'her relief at being given permission not to "let go" is almost palpable'. Having been asked to speak on this 'new model' to groups of bereavement workers around Britain, my impression has been that what I have told them has not been news to their own inner intuition, but they had never heard it publicly legitimated before. They were caught between their own experience and what they perceived as a 'clinical lore' of letting go, cutting ties, moving on, in which they had been trained.

Clinical lore speaks of 'the grief process'. By this is usually meant that grief is not an illness, a state from which one recovers in order to return to the pre-bereavement state, but a process that changes you irrevocably. Now this notion could be compatible with the deceased moving from being with us in the flesh to becoming a group ancestor and/or internalized within the individual mourner, but typically the idea is that the mourner is changed back into a single person, as in the depiction of widowhood as a process of transition from wife to widow to woman. You shift from being an attached person to an unattached autonomous individual, once more able to make new relationships.

Clinical lore posits, basically, one 'grief process', from attachment via emotional pain to autonomy. This implies a common pilgrimage for all bereaved persons, linking them with other pilgrims on the path of bereavement. 'Psychological models construct an imagined wider community of like minded individuals amongst whom the bereaved person can feel at home, symbolically aligning his or her biography with that of other members of the imagined community of the bereaved, who ultimately rejoin the world of the living' (Seale 1998: 198). Clinical lore thus encourages bereaved people not into permanent communion with the dead but into temporary communion with the bereaved. We could analyse this in van Gennepian terms as a transitional, liminal phase, undergirded not by religious ritual but by psychological theory. Unfortunately, as Silverman (1986) and Cline (1996) have pointed out, the liminal identity of widow is a stigmatized one in our society, so is not easily embraced. Undoubtedly, however, many people find a sense of security in belonging to the imagined community of the bereaved: they are not alone, it will not go on for ever.

The revolution

Both the consensus among theorists and clinical lore, however, are changing. Thomas Kuhn (1962) has argued that science develops through 'normal' and 'revolutionary' phases. Normal science accepts a basic paradigm, for example Newton's laws of motion, and on the basis of this thousands of experiments and empirical studies are performed. Findings that challenge the basic paradigm are dismissed as due to faulty equipment or poor methodology. But with time the rogue findings mount up and become more difficult to ignore, though ignored they continue to be because so many professional reputations have been built on the old paradigm. Then comes the revolution. A few key articles gather together all the rogue findings and show that they, as well as all the 'normal' findings, are better explained by a new paradigm. The discipline is in turmoil for a while, before settling down to the next stage of 'normal science'. Such turmoil, I would argue, has characterized the field of bereavement since the late 1980s.

There were two brands of revolutionary. The first were not scholars, but certain people who had themselves been bereaved. Clinical lore relies heavily on studies of prematurely bereaved widows (e.g. Marris 1958; Parkes and Weiss 1983; Parkes 1986), but some younger widows and some bereaved in other circumstances found the conventional wisdom did not apply to them. Many parents who had lost a child could not leave their dead child out of their lives or see future children replacing the dead one. After 10 or 20 years of effective functioning in society, they would still say things such as 'We've got three children, one of whom has died' or 'Once a bereaved parent, always a bereaved parent'. Some prematurely bereaved widows resented the implication that finding a new husband was the only sure evidence of their grief being resolved. Rather than memories of their husband fading, some effectively functioning widows reported the opposite process – at first they were too shocked to remember much, but then began to recall and enjoy more and more memories, leading to a richer rather than an attenuated sense of their dead husband. Though this process is described in texts such as Parkes (1986: 88), such women did not always find clinicians validating such experiences. Many bereaved parents and widows belong to self-help groups such as The Compassionate Friends and The National Association of Widows that distrust theories and experts who are not themselves bereaved.

The other revolutionaries were scholars who were researching other forms of loss than premature loss of a spouse. Articles that reviewed the rapidly mounting body of research found that much of it did not fit the conventional tie-breaking wisdom. Goin *et al.* (1979), Rubin (1984), White (1988) and Stroebe *et al.* (1992) all wrote of continuing attachment to the deceased as normal and healthy. The effect of the revolution may be seen in a small but significant shift from the first (1983) to the second (1991) edition of William Worden's popular textbook *Grief Counselling and Grief Therapy*. Worden describes four 'tasks' of mourning, originally defining the fourth task as 'withdrawing emotional energy from the deceased and reinvesting it in another relationship'. In the second edition (1991: 16), Worden says that he still believes this to be true but that it is easily misunderstood, so he now prefers to say that the task for the counsellor is 'not to help the bereaved give up their relationship with the deceased, but to . . . find an appropriate place for the dead in their emotional lives'. But he still maintains that this 'is hindered by holding on to the past attachment rather than going on and forming new ones'.

In the meantime, unreconstructed Worden, unreconstructed Freud even, is still being taught to the general public. One introductory leaflet about bereavement and counselling, by no means untypical, acknowledges that people grieve in different ways yet still asserts that:

> An important aspect of bereavement counselling is to help people work towards making a healthy emotional withdrawal from the deceased person and to feel comfortable reinvesting their emotion elsewhere.
> (*A Journey Through Bereavement*, North West Hospice, 1996)

No mention here of 'finding an appropriate place for the dead'. So, we are in the middle of a revolution, but it is taking time in some bereavement care organizations for the message to get through to the troops. In others, the troops have been quietly disobeying orders for a while now, with the result that it is taking some time for the revolution to get through to the generals.

Where is the revolution heading? There seem to be three strands of post-revolutionary research. The first, represented by the *Continuing Bonds* volume (Klass *et al.* 1996), emphasizes the inner representations of the deceased held by bereaved individuals and the roles these may play in the grief process. Many questions remain to be researched here concerning the relationship of inner representations to emotional states, physical health and length of mourning. In a word, we know that bonds continue, but is this necessarily good for people and if so what are the mechanisms? The second research strand is interested less in individual psychology and more in the role played by the dead within society as a whole, in collective representations of the dead and the role of collective memory (Middleton and Edwards 1990). Much of this research would not define itself as 'bereavement research', but – with ethnic identity and ethnic conflict a major issue at the turn of the millennium – there is increasing interest in how groups use images of the past in order to represent themselves to themselves and others. I have tried in this book to highlight that research can legitimately go in this direction, as well as in the more conventional direction – for bereavement researchers – of individual psychology. The third strand disputes that there has actually been a revolution. Thus Parkes (1998a, 1998b) locates Klass, Silverman and Nickman's *Continuing Bonds* volume within psycho-social transition theory, arguing that it adds little that is new. Silverman herself has suggested that her book represents evolution within a paradigm rather than a paradigm change.[4] The revolution may yet be incorporated into previous paradigms.

Why now?

If I, and Parkes, are correct that knowledge of continuing bonds with the dead has been around throughout the twentieth century, why is it only at the end of the century that it is moving from the background into the foreground? Why is it only now that so many bereaved people and grief counsellors seem free to acknowledge and validate these bonds? Is there anything in the wider context of culture and ideas that enables this shift?

Stroebe *et al.* (1992) offer a helpful start, by identifying Victorian romanticism, twentieth-century modernism and end-of-century postmodernism as cultural contexts in which grief theories have arisen. Stroebe *et al.* list efficiency, reason, goal directedness and faith in progress as key tenets of cultural modernism. People, like the bereaved, in a state of intense emotionality need to be helped back to effective functioning as quickly as possible; hence the need to 'work through' grief in order to return to normal.

I would add that faith in progress is associated with looking to the future and to the young, rather than to the old and by extension to the ancestors. Who wants to ask the ancestors for advice in a forward looking society? It is the living and the young who have the technical expertise and the vigour that are so highly valued, leaving the old and the dead on the scrap heap. Mourners are thus advised to leave the dead behind. As described in Chapter 1, this is amplified by Protestantism and secularism, both of which find it hard to articulate ways of relating to the dead other than learning from their example – though their example is not always valued in a society that looks to the future rather than to the past. Add to this the individualism that finds it hard to conceive of a community of the living let alone of the dead and we see that any role for the dead that does remain is likely to be within the private experience of the individual – except at those times of war or crisis in which the communal dead are necessary in order to define group identity and boost morale. The 'product' of grief, according to modernistic theory, is the archetypal western individual: self-sufficient, free of all ties and only then able to choose new ties with other individuals on a contractual basis. Certainly not a person who is tied, for good or ill, to an enduring community, whether of the living or of the dead.

It would be particularly useful to know more about ideas and theories of bereavement in countries such as Japan and other Asian societies, which, though fully embracing modernism's efficiency, reason, goal directedness and faith in progress, have been little affected by the Protestantism, secularism and individualism that should, perhaps, be more accurately identified as western rather than modern. I hypothesize such cultures would encourage bereaved people to return to emotional stability as quickly as possible (so they can return to being fully efficient at work), yet grief will result not in the dead being left behind but in their construction as family ancestors. This was the case 30 years ago in Japan (Yamamoto *et al.* 1969); more recently, it seems that the Japanese exercise more choice over which of the family dead they will venerate. Emotional attachment, rather than formal family relationship, is increasingly the determining factor, which seems to represent a degree of westernization.[5]

Stroebe *et al.* (1992) contrast twentieth-century modernism with nineteenth-century romanticism.

> To grieve was to signal the significance of the relationship, and the depth of one's own spirit. Dissolving the bond with the deceased would ... make a sham of a spiritual commitment and undermine one's sense of living a meaningful life ... Valor was found in sustaining these bonds, despite a broken heart.
> (Stroebe *et al.* 1992: 1208)

Clearly there had to be a rejection of romanticism, at least among the (largely male) intelligentsia who produced western grief theories, if Freud's idea of working through the pain of grief in order to become once again a free individual was to take root. Stroebe *et al.* argue that the evidence of continuing bonds with the dead in the twentieth century (Chapters 2–4) indicates that at the level of individual experience romanticism is by no means a thing of the past. Many widows, for example, are torn between the advice of friends to move on and their feeling that this would be to betray their love for their husband. But such experiences were not taken seriously by modernism and its theories. Stroebe *et al.*'s analysis is compatible with that of Ariès (1974; 1981), who argues that today the old Victorian obsession with loss of the other conflicts with the more recent urge to hide death and forget the dead.

Stroebe *et al.* (1992: 1210) suggest that grief theories are now becoming postmodern. Along with postmodern trends elsewhere that undermine overarching 'metanarratives' and emphasize diversity of voice, so both theorists and practitioners are now recognizing in public (they may long have felt this in private) that there is no one way to grieve. Holding on may now be talked of alongside letting go. I entirely agree that it would be hard for thinking about bereavement to be insulated from the wider trend against universal theories and toward diversity. But does contemporary culture make it easier to speak specifically of continuing bonds with the dead? Possibly so, and to explore why we must return to the key aspects of modernism that underlay the breaking ties view. Efficiency and goal directedness are still central to the operation of modern economies, so the requirement to return mourners to emotional stability as quickly as possible remains. More relevant is what is happening to the modern virtues of progress and rationality and to the western virtues of Protestantism and secularism.

Although it can be argued that the idea of ever-continuing progress sustained severe setbacks throughout the twentieth century (for example, the First World War, mass unemployment, fascism, the Holocaust and so forth), in the last third of the century it seems to have been questioned even more.[6] Vietnam, Watergate, the environmental crisis, Generation X, all these signal a loss of faith in the grand narratives of modernity and assured progress. Associated with this has been a growing nostalgia for the past, and an interest in how pre-modern societies lived and died before they got messed up by western industrialism. A culture that is looking backwards is more likely to take bonds with the dead seriously.

Postmodern times are hard times for rationality. It could be argued that there is now a popular culture of sentimentality (Anderson and Mullen 1998), a celebration of Venusian female virtues over Martian male ones (Gray 1993), that enables emotions, including the emotions of grief, to be valued more highly. Yet nobody is disputing emotional stability as an ultimate goal for mourners if society, economy and families are to continue to function.

In modernism, people did not acknowledge their relationships with the dead because (1) they did not seem rational, people might think you were mad, and (2) four centuries of Protestantism had banned relations with the dead. But much of the English-speaking world has become secular, and children no longer attend the Sunday schools where their predecessors had learned the Protestant ban, whose effect is consequently much reduced.[7] Toward the end of the millennium, along with environmental awareness has come a less wholehearted infatuation with science and technology: we need them, not least to fix the environmental mess, but they are perceived to have caused the mess in the first place. It is in this context of scepticism about science and rationality that many people are prepared to explore ideas that previously would have been dismissed as cranky: abduction by aliens, alternative healing, near-death experiences – and sensing the presence of the dead. Popular culture is losing its Protestantism, glances backwards and sideways (to other cultures) as well as forwards to an uncertain future, and has become more open to the apparently irrational, rendering it respectable for the first time in a century to speak openly about sensible contemporary people bonding with the dead.

Protestantism alone did not have the power to prevent relating to the dead. The nineteenth century was, after all, one in which Protestantism was embraced by many middle- and upper-class women who also embraced their dead. But there was always a tension between looking forward to the family reunions of which romanticism spoke, and looking forward to heavenly bliss in the company of the Lord Jesus of which evangelical Protestantism spoke (Ariès 1981; McDannell and Lang 1988). Evangelical mourners could live with this tension because the powerful emphasis their religion placed on family love resonated with the romanticism that spoke of family reunion in heaven.

Last, but possibly not least, gender. I have hinted above that modern notions of rationality have largely been promoted by men and that the notion of the autonomous individual is distinctly male. Research (biological, psychological and sociological) has demonstrated that women are typically better at intuiting the feelings of others and connecting to other people, are less competitive and less willing to inflict harm. Even those who dispute the biological or universal nature of such findings, acknowledge that the nineteenth and twentieth centuries have witnessed the ascription of these connective virtues to women rather than to men. Hence, the mourner who speedily leaves grief behind and returns to personal autonomy is typically a male. Modernistic grief theory pathologizes the prolonged emotionality and reluctance to loosen ties with the beloved that characterizes many female mourners. It may be no coincidence that twentieth-century grief theories have been challenged at precisely the time that women have begun to articulate their own voice. The vast majority of counsellors and popular writers on bereavement are women, many working and writing out of a personal experience of loss that simply does not fit the male model of letting go (Simonds and Rothman 1992). Many are at pains to say that grief does not end. Women's rediscovered voice makes it easier to speak of the importance of bonding over individual autonomy, in death as well as in life, for men as well as for women.

Summary

Since Freud, twentieth-century theories have concentrated on how bereaved people must 'work through' grief in order eventually to 'detach' themselves from the one to whom in life they had been attached. Some theorists have also included the process by which the deceased is internalized – sometimes seen as merely a temporary precursor to detachment, sometimes as a long-term alternative to it. Nevertheless, a clinical lore developed that required the breaking of affectional bonds with the deceased. This fitted the requirements of an efficiency-oriented, secular society composed of autonomous individuals. By the 1980s, however, this goal of 'letting go' was being challenged, both by bereaved people and by researchers. Voicing this challenge has been made possible by a number of cultural changes in society at large: the shift in authority from expert to consumer, the increasing confidence of women to challenge male experts, the postmodern celebration of diversity over monolithic theories of human behaviour, the undermining of the notion of progress and a new openness to the paranormal.

Further reading

Fraley, C. and Shaver, P. (forthcoming) Theories of grief in contemporary research, in M. Stroebe, W. Stroebe, R. Hansson and H. Schut (eds) *New Handbook of Bereavement*. Washington, DC: American Psychological Association Press.

Parkes, C.M. (forthcoming) An historical overview of the scientific study of bereavement, in M. Stroebe, W. Stroebe, R. Hansson and H. Schut (eds) *New Handbook of Bereavement*. Washington, DC: American Psychological Association Press.

Silverman, P. and Klass, D. (1996) Introduction: what's the problem? in D. Klass, P.R. Silverman and S.L. Nickman (eds) *Continuing Bonds*: New Understandings of Grief. Bristol, PA and London: Taylor & Francis.

Stroebe, M., Gergen, M.M., Gergen, K.J., Stroebe, W. (1992) Broken hearts or broken bonds: love and death in historical perspective. *American Psychologist*, 47: 1205–12. (Reprinted in D. Klass *et al.* (eds) (1996) *Continuing Bonds*.)

Questions

1 Discuss the role of internalizing the dead in the writings of Freud, Bowlby, or Parkes.
2 What is your own experience of being taught about bereavement, and when was this? What were you taught about 'letting go'? What is the relationship between your own experience of loss and what you were taught?
3 What do you understand by the term 'the grief process'?
4 Does your gender or your religious faith affect your understanding of how the living relate to the dead?

Notes

1 See Peskin (1993) and Stroebe *et al.* (1993) for competing interpretations of Bowlby's work on this point.

2 The term 'clinical lore' comes from Wortman and Silver (1989).

3 For the record, I would now make the following clarifications and modifications to the article: (1) The model adds to the diversity of descriptions of how people grieve. I do not intend to replace one grand theory with another. (2) As will be clear from Part I of this book, I would not now say that all bereaved people *need* to incorporate the dead into their ongoing lives. Some do. Some do not. For this reason, I am unhappy nowadays talking about incorporating the dead as grief's 'goal' or 'purpose'. (3) It is typically more important that the story which people create about the dead be *shared* than that it be accurate. It is in the sharing of the story that the social reality of the dead is constructed and maintained. There are, however, certain circumstances in which the story, if it is to be shared, must be accurate; there are other circumstances where the story cannot be shared and may need to remain private. (4) I do not think there is any question of talking about the dead being an *alternative* to expressing the emotions of loss. Indeed, they often go together. To give two examples: talking about the dead often brings forth tears, and facing up to problematic emotions may be necessary before an enduring story about the deceased can be constructed. (5) I am now more aware of the diversity of techniques and strategies that go under the generic name of 'bereavement counselling'.

4 She suggested this at the Bereavement Research Forum, Oxford, 17 November 1998.

5 Dennis Klass, personal communication.

6 The idea of personal growth – everlasting progress in the personal sphere – is, however, booming, and has had a major influence on popular books on bereavement. 'You can grow through grief' is the basic message.

7 I speak here only of Britain and other historically Protestant European countries, along with Australia and New Zealand. The United States (and of course Northern Ireland) is still buoyantly religious and – in many quarters – vigorously Protestant.

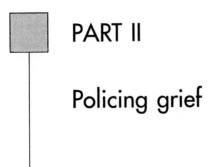

PART II

Policing grief

Introduction to Part II

On the shoulders of mourners falls the task of integrating the dead into society, though they may receive little thanks for this – witness the criticism in Britain, first from intellectuals and then from others, of how people mourned Diana, Princess of Wales. This brings us to my second theme: how does society regulate bereavement, how does it control and instruct the bereaved how to think, feel and behave?

To the best of my knowledge, there is no society – apart from in some ways our own – in which bereaved people are left to their own devices. Paul Rosenblatt, who probably knows more about grief across cultures than anyone else on earth, concludes, 'I know of no society in which the emotions of bereavement are not shaped and controlled, for the sake of the deceased, the bereaved person, or others' (1997: 36). Traditional funeral rituals and mourning practices regulate, channel and elicit the emotions of mourners, often, it has to be said, in ways not to their taste. Though it is sometimes imagined that in non-industrial societies, traditional rituals enable people to express their grief freely and naturally, the evidence is to the contrary: the expression of grief by mourners in such societies is often more, not less, subject to socially accepted rules than is the case in Anglo-American society.

In many societies, such as rural Greece and early modern England, certain classes of people (e.g. older women, the poor) were expected to keen and mourn for people they did not themselves personally grieve. In many societies, the dramatically greater grief expressed by women suggests not just that they feel more, but that they are required to mourn on behalf of men, ritually expressing men's grief as well as their own. In other societies, the expression of grief is discouraged (Wikan 1988), not least because it is considered that if the departed become aware of the loud wailing of survivors they will become distressed and want to return to earth to comfort them, thus impeding their progress to the next world. We see something of this in the study by Scheper-Hughes (1990: 559) of child death among the urban poor of northeast Brazil: 'It is a grave sin for a mother to cry for the first 60 days after her baby's death', said Dona Marlene, 'because their mother's tears will make the road from earth to heaven slippery and he will lose his footing and fall.' In none of these societies are mourners left to follow a 'natural grief process'. Grief is regulated, controlled, patrolled, policed.

So, when I write of 'policing' grief, I do not yearn for an emotional anarchy in which controlling grief's unruly feelings is unnecessary. All societies police grief, but the goals, methods and approaches of this control have varied considerably, and indeed are a matter of considerable debate in contemporary western societies. Part 2 provides a sketch map of the current debates, and an introduction to the politics of grief.

Regulating grief

Mourners are rarely left alone in their grief. The criticisms they often face ('You should have got over him by now', 'I'm concerned you never shed any tears for her', 'Why did you get so upset at the death of a princess you never met?') indicate that people consider there to be norms for bereaved people to follow, and that these norms are by no means always followed and/or there is not agreement over them. One of Durkheim's key interests was how society controls and regulates what he called 'the passions' or what we might today term emotion.

Passionate emotions may follow bereavement, but may not. (I may not have loved my wife and may be pleased that I can now take up with my mistress.) But often the emotions of grief are raw, unexpected and frightening – both to the individual and to onlookers – and that is why they get policed.[1] If Durkheim is right that passions cannot be left to run their course without social regulation, then this explains why all societies have rules for how the emotions of grief are to be displayed and handled.

Thus far, we might imagine grief to be like a steam engine, powerful and ready to explode unless regulated and channelled. But Durkheimian anthropologists emphasize that social rules of mourning do not just regulate naturally existing emotion. They also impose duties of mourning, even on those who otherwise feel little. Like many a play or movie, funeral and mourning rituals may not only allow existing emotion to be expressed, they can also evoke emotion de novo. Grief is performed, evoked by social context as much as bursting out from within; clear rules typically exist for its performance (Davies 1997: 44–8). Mourners may be required to mourn, whatever they do or do not personally feel about the deceased. There are emotional scripts (Sarbin 1986a) that have to be followed. Such scripts may be found, for example, in Susan Hill's (1977) novel *In the Springtime of the Year*, a book frequently recommended to bereaved people in the UK. Set in a traditional English village, 19-year-old Ruth loses her husband Ben in a freak accident. Ruth and Ben's mother, Dora, grieve in different ways, and Ruth muses on the expectations on both of them at the funeral:

> Dora Bryce was walking unsteadily, clinging to her husband's arm, and to Alice on the other side, and so it was around her that people gathered, for they knew what to do with a woman who wept or fainted, who behaved in the way that seemed right, seemed customary . . . [That night, Ruth] listened to the keening of Dora Bryce, it came to her as clearly as if there were no walls to the house. It was a terrible noise, she was ashamed of the woman for making it, and ashamed of herself, because she could not.
>
> (Hill 1977: 55–6)

Grief is surrounded by expectations, which bereaved people may be all too aware of, and may themselves have internalized. But, as Ruth found, that does not mean that everyone mourns as prescribed.

At the time of writing, many bereaved people feel they are expected to keep quiet about their grief, at least after the first few weeks. But in the bereavement literature that has proliferated toward the end of the twentieth century, there is another expectation: that bereaved people should express their grief. Though this literature typically portrays silence as imposed and expression as natural, a sociological or anthropological perspective (Armstrong 1987) sees both silence and talk as socially imposed, though by different groups. There can be a requirement to speak as well as a requirement to keep silent, an expectation to weep as well an expectation as keep a stiff upper lip. It is heresy to say this in those circles for whom a cardinal article of faith is that the expression of grief is natural and healthy, whereas silence is imposed and psychologically damaging. But all I am observing in our own society is what for a hundred years anthropologists have been observing in non-western societies.

To mourn or not to mourn?

There is at present in the western world considerable disarray over the regulation or policing of grief.[2] It is widely believed by bereavement workers that the more formal mourning rituals of previous times and of other cultures provided clear guidelines for grieving. As The Compassionate Friends leaflet *Bereaved Parents and the Professional* (no date) puts it 'Our Society today has lost the mourning rituals once routinely accepted, that helped families in their sadness.' Without such rituals, mourners are left without guidance, in a state of what Durkheim termed anomie, that is, without norms. Yet, as we shall see in Chapter 7, twentieth-century people chose to give up traditional mourning, for very good reasons. They, especially upper-class women, did not want to be swathed in black for months or years, they wanted freedom to grieve as felt right to them as individuals. Much contemporary literature on grief asserts that everyone grieves differently and that there cannot be rules. Hill's novel is a poignant account of one young woman's determination to go through grief her way, not the way traditionally expected in her village. So we now have a situation where the literature on bereavement bemoans the lack of policing that traditional mourning rituals provided, yet at the same time promotes the idea that grief should not be policed but should be allowed to express itself naturally.

When we listen to bereaved people, it is clear they are often tossed this way and that. Sometimes they feel they are expected to grieve in ways that do not feel right to them as individuals; maybe they want to express their grief but their family disapproves of this. Sometimes the mourning rules they grew up with, for example contain your feelings and grieve in private, do not match what they read in magazines, that it is healthy to let feelings out. The professional advice they receive may not fit lay advice. Or the time scales for grief differ. The result is that their grief is either over- or under-policed.

Over-regulation

Columnist Virginia Ironside, from her own experience of grief on losing her father, passionately advocates that each bereavement is unique to the individual and one of the added pains of bereavement is other people:

> The wretched thing about all this is that if you do grieve, people are nagging at you to cheer up; but if you don't grieve people are nagging at you to grieve. They are comfortable with some grief, but not too much. They are comfortable with good cheer – but again, not too much ... We each have our own ways of coping and if keeping objects helps, then keep; if chucking helps, then chuck. Psychologists would have us believe that those who keep everything are trying to deny that anything has happened; and guess what they say about people who chuck everything out? Yup. They, too, are denying.
>
> (Ironside 1996: 85, 110)

Ironside does admit that bereaved people can be very touchy – whatever the would-be comforter says is likely to be wrong.

A common complaint, usually from women, of over-regulation concerns the expression of emotion. One widow described her husband: 'He said, "Come on now, pull yourself together; you've done really well so far, don't break down now." I couldn't even cry at home after that' (Littlewood

1992: 120). The other most common complaint, also typically from women, is that other people (women as well as men) expect her to have got over her grief long before she actually has. Silverman's (1986) middle aged American widows were distressed that, though friends and family were very supportive in the first few weeks, thereafter the expectation was that the widow would get back to normal and should begin dating within a few months. Mutual help groups (Chapter 11) claim to provide a haven from such expectations.

One might be tempted to argue (compare Simonds and Rothman 1992; Cline 1996) that the policing of grief is essentially patriarchal, involving the policing of females by males. It may, however, be emotionality, impaired functioning and reminders of death, rather than women, that are the targets of social regulation. Much of the policing is done by females – by family and friends who do not want to be reminded that their husbands or their children could also die – and some of those who feel over-controlled are males. It may simply be that there are many more widows than widowers, and that bereaved mothers – having carried the baby in the womb – are more likely than fathers to sense that the loss of a child is a loss of themselves. In other words, there is simply more female grief around, but when males grieve deeply they are just as likely to be policed, as in the following case.

A newspaper article titled 'One Year On: the terrible legacy of Oklahoma' (*The Guardian* 18 April 1996), describes the conflicting expectations between professionals and bereaved people concerning how long it would take for grief to subside following the Oklahoma City bombing in which over 150 people died:

> Counsellors are surprised how many 'are still mired in grief and anger'.
>
> Bud Welch, 56, doesn't want to hear any more talk of 'closure'. He lost his daughter Julie, 23, in the blast. 'When they imploded the building, they said it was for closure. When the last three bodies were found, they said it would help closure. When they laid the grass [on the site of the blast] they talked about closure. That word is so damned over-used. That just doesn't happen. There is no closure.'
>
> Welch has visited the site every day since the bombing, sometimes more than once. Seeing the endless stream of people who come to place makeshift crosses and stuffed animals and flowers and messages in the wire fence around the ground where the Murrah Building stood, cheers him up. Often he strikes up conversations with them. 'It gives me a chance to brag about my daughter. She wouldn't permit me to brag about her when she was alive.'

Like many bereaved parents, Welch finds congruent expectations among fellow mourners that he fails to find among professional 'experts'. With fellow mourners, he finds people willing to hear the story of his daughter.

Under-regulation

If some bereaved people complain of having their grief policed inappropriately, whether by friends, family or professionals, others suffer because they do not have enough guidance and knowledge about grief. They experience under-regulation (which Durkheim (1952) termed anomie). Due to the widespread norm that grief should be expressed privately (Chapter 8), adults often take care not to display their grief, not even to other family members. Indeed, many parents feel children should be protected from grief. So children grow up without having observed adults' grief or how they deal with it. As a result, many bereaved people in the modern West are surprised and disturbed by the emotions they feel, to the extent they feel they are going mad. Bereavement workers and mutual help groups often assure the newly bereaved that intense feelings – such as guilt, anger, or aroused sexuality – are perfectly normal. Mutual help groups and counselling (Chapter 11) educate new members into what bereavement entails.

Bereaved people may therefore seek support from agencies and mutual help groups *both* because they are policed too rigidly by friends and relatives and want somewhere to express their feelings and tell the story of the deceased, *and* because they are in the dark about their emotional responses and want guidance and reassurance. Over- and under-regulation together account for many referrals to bereavement groups and agencies. These two problems have been receiving increasing attention in bereavement literature over the past three decades, but this is the first book that specifically analyses them. This is because many (not all) bereavement books see grief as essentially a natural psychological process that resides within the individual, a process that may be merely supported or impeded by social context. By contrast, I suggest that the interpersonal processes of integration and regulation can be *as* important as any intra-personal processes.

Self-regulation

Much of the policing of grief is self-policing.[3] People read books that provide *descriptions* of grief and read them as *prescriptions* – because they want guidelines, they want to know how long their pain will last. Many bereaved people are concerned to know 'how they are getting on', which is one reason for the ease with which self-help and autobiographical grief books sell. By comparing themselves with others further along in 'the grief process', or by locating themselves in terms of stage theories, bereaved people gain an idea of where they themselves have got to and whether their own grief is 'normal'. In addition, bereaved people learn what things to say and what emotions to reveal (as with the widow who learned not to cry in front of her husband). Whereas the upper-class Victorian widow was doing the right thing so long as she wore mourning dress for the correct period (with her veil conveniently hiding her actual feelings), the twentieth-century widow is altogether more naked. The gaze of self and others is no longer on her dress or even her behaviour, but on her feelings, which are much harder to assess, still less to timetable. So anxiety about 'Am I feeling the right things? Am I going mad?' escalates. 'The grief process' has replaced traditional mourning as the main construct by which grief is structured (Wambach 1985), but it is never clear quite where in the grief process one has got to.

Contemporary bereavement is a matter of self-monitoring, assisted by advice from family and friends, bereavement books, counsellors and mutual help groups. In this, bereavement is like contemporary marriage and child-rearing in which partners and parents are always asking how well they are doing, consulting the baby books to see if their child's development is above or below average, consulting their therapist to get the most out of their marriage. In fact, bereavement is like the rest of contemporary life, a reflexive process of checking that one is doing okay (Giddens 1991). Beck and Beck-Gernsheim (1995) argue that in a detraditionalized society, couples have to make up their own rules, for example about the division of labour in the home, so that the normal course of love is somewhat chaotic. At long last, feudalism has been replaced by democracy in personal relations between men and women as well as in politics – order is no longer given, but has to be constantly negotiated and created by the partners. This is liberating, but much harder work than accepting given roles. We might say the same about grief: with de-traditionalization, grief is even more chaotic than ever, especially within families. The democratization of grief, like the democratization of marriage, may be an advance in freedom, but the flipside is an increase in chaos, anomie and uncertainty. The psychological construct of 'the grief process' has been introduced in order to do something to order the chaos of grief, which is why the debate (Chapters 6 and 9) about what precisely constitutes 'the grief process' is more than academic.

Some caveats

Since the early nineteenth century, the ordinary police force has been a specialist and clearly identified occupational group, but I hope it is clear by now that I am not reserving the policing of grief for those who are professionally involved in bereavement work. Primarily families, but also employers, friends, themselves and only finally professional bereavement workers all police the bereaved. Often, bereavement counselling provides a free space from over-heavy policing by families.

Durkheim was more interested in the social functions of human behaviour than in the meanings that individuals give to their behaviour and this is reflected in my emphasis on regulating or policing grief. When I write about families or professionals policing grief, I am speaking of the functions, the consequences, of their actions. I am emphatically not talking about the actors' intentions. Bereavement work, for example, may function to police grief or it may function to liberate clients from over-policing; the *motives* of bereavement workers may be entirely different, chiefly the concern to ameliorate the manifest suffering of their clients.

When people refer to 'the grief police', they typically do so perjoratively. One hospice worker wrote to me following the death of his wife: 'I was warned by my daughter not to let the Grief Police get at me.' During what was effectively a week of required mourning, those who did not wish to mourn Princess Diana referred scathingly to 'the grief police' and Britain having become 'a police state'. But any civilized society needs policing, and it is in this more neutral sense that I speak of policing the disturbingly anti-social emotions of grief. Part 2 charts the way this policing has developed historically and is currently under contentious review.

Notes

1 At this point I agree with those who argue that grief has the characteristics of mental disorder.
2 My concept of policing has similarities to Foucault's (1973, 1977) notion of 'the gaze' and of institutions that discipline their members.
3 A link might be made here to the work of Norbert Elias (1978, 1982), who argues that over the past millennium the civilizing process has entailed a long-term shift from lack of control of bodily and sexual functions, to control of them by others (for example, by shaming), to self-control.

7 Guidelines for grief: historical background

Grief is itself a medicine.

(William Cowper, 1731–1800)

When I am dead, my dearest,
sing no sad songs for me

(Christina Rossetti, 1830–94)

This chapter sketches selected aspects of the historical background to contemporary mourning and its regulation.

The cult of melancholy

Houlbrooke's (1998: 221) description of upper-class sixteenth- and seventeenth-century England will sound familiar to many contemporary readers: 'Excessive grief was generally deprecated. To surrender to one's feelings showed a lack of faith, reason, self-control, even a perverse wilfulness. Not to feel grief at all, however, was unnatural.' At the same time, there was increasing interest in personality and experience, as found in new poetic forms, the introspective diary, intimate biography, the development of letter-writing skills and the novel. All this entailed a more reflexive self-awareness about mourning and melancholy. Indeed, at the beginning of the seventeenth century a positive cult of melancholy flourished in both music and poetry; jilted young men were expected to go around with long faces writing self-pitying couplets . *Ye Sacred Muses*, William Byrd's exquisitely sad elegy for Thomas Tallis, plaintively repeating 'Tallis is dead, music has died', articulates both personal and communal loss on the death of that generation's finest composer.

Puritans, concerned that intense grief might manifest itself in wanting to pray for the departed, a Romish and iniquitous practice, were handicapped in finding religious expressions of grief. Grief was expressed instead in secular literary forms, which by the eighteenth century included graveyard poetry, a flourishing popular genre of which Gray's famous *Elegy in a Country Churchyard* of 1745 is a late example and only one among thousands (Draper 1967). Draper observes that reason thinks in terms of abstractions and generalizations, emotions in terms of the specific and the particular. Emotional graveyard poetry explored the particular place in which the body lay, giving rise to detailed descriptions of nature. This, Draper argues, is a significant source of the romantic interest in nature; funeral elegies elaborated on precisely the nocturnal atmosphere that led later to the construction of grottoes and gothic ruins. Whereas it is normally argued that romanticism helped foster the death culture of the Victorian era, Draper suggests that romanticism itself drew on the need to speak of mortality and mourning in a culture that eschewed grand requiem masses. In turn, this helped create the Victorian cult of the cemetery. This cult was, of course, highly developed in Catholic countries, such as France, as much as in Protestant countries. But it may be significant that the romantic association of the grave with nature is specific to Protestant Germany, Scandinavia and Britain, whereas Catholic France, Italy and Spain built their cemeteries to resemble mini-cities.[1]

Today, the English may have long lost the cult of melancholy, but with a cremation rate of 70 per cent and with most people living in towns, the romantic idea of being laid finally to rest in an English country churchyard still appeals, even if few are entitled to it. In Scandinavia, burial in a cemetery in the primeval forest remains an option for many.

Enlightened sympathy

The architect Sir John Soane was devastated by the death of his wife in 1815; he received numerous letters from friends criticizing him for overindulging his grief and exhorting him to keep busy and to remarry. They expressed exasperation at his lack of willingness to master his grief (Gittings 1997). We can see in this advice the guidelines for grief of two centuries earlier, but their advice also reflected Adam Smith's theory of condolence, published in his *Theory of Moral Sentiments* (1759/1976). Smith argued that the basis of social solidarity is sympathy, sharing the feelings of others. It is the responsibility of the sufferer to try to reduce his feelings to those of his comforters, who in turn should make efforts to raise their feelings to meet his – only then can sympathy be given and received. Soane's friends were annoyed because they were making an effort but he was not. Smith's theory clearly shows condolence to be a social interaction with rules that both parties must follow if comfort is to be given and received. Conducted sensitively, 'society and conversation, therefore, are the most powerful remedies for restoring the mind to its tranquillity' (Smith 1759/1976: I.i.4.10; see also Schor 1994).

Durkheim (1912/1965), another thinker in the Enlightenment tradition but writing a century and a half later, propounded a similar theory. Aboriginals who are not themselves personally bereaved may nevertheless weep or even lacerate themselves, which Durkheim interpreted as their way of aligning their behaviour and feelings with those who really were bereaved and thus generating solidarity. Like Smith's conversational condolence, acting and feeling as if you yourself were bereaved links you to the truly bereaved, generates fellow feeling and is the root of social solidarity (see also Huntington and Metcalf 1979: 28–34).

Observation reveals this kind of sympathy to be common today. People feel sad for those who have experienced a loss with which they can identify, even if the comforter never even met the deceased. When in such a case the comforter says 'I'm sorry', she may not be lying: even though she did not originally feel sorry that the person whom she had never met had died, she has nevertheless manipulated her emotions so that now she does indeed feel at least a little bit sorry, in order to show solidarity with and sympathy for the mourner. In September 1997, millions felt sorry for Princess Diana's two boys, aged 12 and 15 years, imagining what it must be like to lose your mother and generating a palpable and nation-wide wave of sympathy and solidarity.

By contrast, today's bereavement literature advises attentive listening but never to presume to say 'I know how you feel'; such a statement may well be incorrect or be perceived to be so by the bereaved person, inducing a sense of alienation from rather than connection with the would-be comforter. Certainly the normal practice of psychodynamic counsellors is to keep their own feelings out of the picture, and they may well need to do this if they are not to be engulfed by the human sorrow they encounter, but this is not how friends, neighbours and colleagues operate.[2] Adam Smith may be nearer the mark when it comes to describing how ordinary people relate to the suffering of others. In offering sympathy (actually showing your feelings), rather than empathy (showing an understanding of how the other person feels), the comforter does his or her best to feel something of what the sufferer feels and this can be appreciated by the sufferer. But the sufferer must be open to this overture, and not – at least in conversation with others – wallow in their suffering, moaning that 'nobody feels like I do' or 'nobody understands', as apparently did Soane.

Some forms of loss make it difficult to express sympathy. Bereaved parents have often reported that other parents with live children do not want the dead child mentioned indefinitely and can be very unhelpful. Blank (1998: 36) has the honesty to admit that she too was like this before her own daughter died. Friends may drop away, but kin are always there – for better or for worse. Blank describes the breakdown in ties of kin that can occur when the bereaved parent wishes to talk about her child yet the relatives cannot stand the constant reminders that their own child too could die. In Adam Smith's terms, it simply is too painful for them to begin to feel even a little of what she feels, so they give up the attempt; in turn, they feel she is not really trying to get on top of her grief. Mutual help groups for bereaved parents are full of mothers who have had this kind of experience and who value the group as an enclave where the child can be talked of and feelings expressed, indefinitely, among people whose feelings already match their own.

VICTORIAN GRIEF AND ITS ECHOES

The high period of Victorian mourning, around 1850–1890, still leaves its echoes, even as we enter the twenty-first century. Twentieth-century mourning (in all social classes) is partly an evolution of certain aspects of upper- and middle-class Victorian mourning, partly a reaction against it. This is the subject of the remainder of this chapter.

From respectability to liberty

Victorian mourning demonstrated the respectability of your family, was a task that largely fell on women and, formally at least, had little to do with how you personally felt about the one who had died (Morley 1971; Taylor 1983). Nevertheless, many Victorian women did enter wholeheartedly into mourning. In an age of patronage in which women could achieve status only by marriage, the rules of mourning may in practice have reflected quite closely the actual grief felt by many women. They had lost not only their husband, but also their status, and possibly any right to financial mainten-ance. But in the higher classes at least, formality reigned. There were clear rules for how long you mourned a spouse, a child, a grandchild, a sibling, a parent, and significantly there was no formal mourning period for a friend, however close you may have been. The wife bore the brunt of mourning for the husband's relatives, she being required to stay at home in mourning while he was allowed to go out and attend social events. Inferiors mourned superiors – workers for their employers, subjects for the sovereign, women for their husbands' relatives – not the other way around. As late as the 1920s, the respectable working class still subjected its members to status-driven mourning:

> A superior servant, a mere girl, married a house painter. Within a year of the event, the husband fell from a ladder and was killed.

The poor little widow bought a cheap black dress and a very simple black straw hat to wear at the funeral. Her former employer, who had much commended this modest outlay, met the girl a few days later swathed in crape, her poor little face only half visible under a hideous widow's bonnet complete with streamers and a veil. Asked why she had made these purchases she explained that her neighbours and relations had made her life unbearable because she did not want to wear widow's weeds, and at last she had to give in. 'They said that if I would not wear a bonnet, *it proved we were never married*,' she sobbed.

(Puckle 1926: 97)

By this time, the middle classes – represented in this story by the girl's employer – had begun to reject the trappings of Victorian mourning. Indeed, Puckle's book is one of a number of the period inveighing against the excesses of Victorian mourning, as his Preface (1926: 5) indicates: 'It is a wholesome sign that a more enlightened public is slowly releasing death from much of its ugly trappings.' He goes on to quote Bacon from 300 years earlier, 'Death, beautiful in itself, is only made terrible by groans and convulsions and a discoloured face, and friends weeping and blacks and obsequies.' Victorian mourning lingered well into the mid-twentieth century among the working and upper classes, but – starting with the middle-classes – the social requirement to mourn in prescribed ways was increasingly rejected in favour of a respect for the privacy of grief and for the right to mourn according to how, and for how long, one wanted to. It is now felt that mourning should reflect personal attachment and inner feeling, which in turn should not be paraded ostentatiously.

As the twentieth century unfolded and women gained more sources of status apart from their husbands, they freed themselves from the respectable obligation to mourn. Indeed, the erosion of Victorian mourning in upper middle-class circles from the 1890s is related to the movement for female emancipation: the suffragettes and the collapse of Victorian mourning have the same inspiration. Grieving and voting could now both be engaged in by women in their own right.

The effect of all this is that socially required mourning has given way to privately experienced grief. Initially experienced as liberation, many critics of the western way of grief (stemming from Gorer's classic book of 1965) now claim that this de-regulation has left mourners without guidelines and in a state of anomie. Critics bemoan the loss of the rituals that once regulated emotion, yet no one now wants to impose rituals regardless of how the individual feels. These same critics therefore advocate personally chosen and individually tailored rituals (e.g. Albery *et al.* 1993). These can provide an opportunity for social support, and validation of one's chosen style of grieving by one's chosen friends.

From spontaneous grief to stoicism

Closely regulated by social convention, Victorian mourning paradoxically also allowed the spontaneous expression of grief, within specified limits (Ariès 1974: ch.3). In much of Europe, though not of Britain, cemetery sculpture came to include nubile and near-naked young women swooning over the grave (Robinson 1995). Painting of the period is replete with grieving individuals, both male and female, revealing inner feelings as much as social convention. Though formal funeral processions were the subject of some paintings, many more showed the distraught individual, as in Thomas Barker's *The Bride of Death* (1838) in which the young husband throws himself on the dead body of his young bride. At the end of the period, Puccini's opera *La Bohème* ends with a similar scene. Both the Romantic movement and (in Britain and North America) the Evangelical revival demanded emotional expression (Jalland 1996: 4–5), though this set up a tension between expressivity and Christian hope. Pious nineteenth-century American diarists controlled the expression of their grief, even in the privacy of a diary, for fear this would imply a lack of faith or that they doubted God's wisdom in taking their beloved (Rosenblatt 1983: 101–2).

By the 1870s and 1880s, however, the age of open expression was waning among the upper classes. Evangelicalism and Romanticism were in decline, accelerated for upper-class males by a public school ethos of manliness and emotional reserve (Jalland 1996), an ethos that percolated down via boys' books and magazines to the middle classes and even to girls (Cadogan and Craig 1976). By the First World War, stoicism had replaced keening as the dominant response to loss. One fictional dead serviceman, via a medium, begged the bereaved not to mourn, for every tear was like torture to dead men:

> Tell the mothers and fathers and sisters and wives to stop crying. No man can stand the sight of tears, the sound of sobs. They feel it much worse here . . . for heaven's sake beg the mourners to stop crying and to cease wearing black clothes.
> (Rutherford 1920: 36, 39, cited in Bourke 1996: 221–1)

I suggested in Chapter 2 that mass bereavement through war tends to lead to the dead being left behind: there are so many of them and there is a war to be fought. By the same token, emotions have to be suppressed if the war effort is to continue, and with multiple loss an emotional switching off may be a natural defence mechanism. When suppression of emotion becomes a national necessity during war, it may have a knock-on effect in the following peace. With the emotional excesses of Victorian mourning already in decline, the First World War accelerated a change that was already under way. Half a century later, an American widow recalled:

Last year he said to me, 'If anything ever happens to me I don't want
you to go to pieces. I want you to act like Jacqueline Kennedy – you
know, very brave and courageous. You've got to have class,' he said. 'I
just don't want screaming and hollering.'

(Glick *et al.* 1974: 60)

A fatalistic attitude to one's own demise is a well-known response in war,
as it is in dangerous occupations such as mining, fishing and steel-making:

Fatalism plays quite a part in my attitude and it may have something
to do with the 1939–1945 war. I was 14 in 1939 and remember shel-
tering under the stairs and underground when the bombers were over
Liverpool. There were one or two near misses and this affected my
choice of the R.A.F. I was too late to fight, but even so flying was quite
a death defying business. (The service slang word 'dicey' derives from
dicing with death in an aeroplane.) I lost one or two friends through
crashes and had a couple of close calls myself.[3]

Another veteran from World War Two who had had a near death experience at Dunkirk and later some gruesome experiences in Normandy, wrote
to me that 'Death is not something to fear, rather it is something to await
with patience and equanimity and finally, rejoice over.' It would seem likely
that this fatalism could apply to death of the other as well as death of the
self. Whereas in peacetime one might rail against God or become engulfed
in self-pity that your husband died of cancer before his time or that your
child died, this was not appropriate in war. Many accepted stoically that it
was a lottery whose son was killed at the front, or whose house received a
direct hit. Knowing you were not the only one whom fate had touched may
also have helped.

A more recent example of fatalistic stoicism was shown in the BBC
television documentary *Alison's Last Mountain*. Alison Hargreaves died
climbing K2, the world's second highest mountain, and the programme
documented the pilgrimage of her husband James Ballard and their two
young children to the foot of the mountain. Ballard, dry-eyed throughout,
later commented that mountaineers see death not as a tragedy but as an
occupational hazard.[4]

But not that many take up genuinely risky sports. Most people in the
modern West now live in historically unprecedented safety. Our children
are not conscripted and sent into battle and, thanks to de-industrialization
and the contemporary obsession with minimizing risk, the numbers engaged
in dangerous occupations are less than ever before. Now we are struck
by the unfairness of accidental or premature death and people can afford
to be emotional. Yet our mores this century have been shaped by both
war and a reaction against Victorian sentimentality; they are not easily
abandoned even though the conditions that shaped them are, thankfully,

long gone. So the stiff upper lip is not so easily shed. This is the historical background against which many contemporary bereavement books are written, urging us to leave behind decades of stoicism and to cry if we want to (e.g. Carmichael 1991; Lendrum and Syme 1992). Such books portray tears as natural and healthy; from the perspective of this chapter, however, they are a product of a time and place, in this case an unprecedently safe world.

In the subculture of dangerous occupations – fishing, mining, ambulance work, the police, the armed services, professional mountaineering – stoicism is resilient, resisting the advice of many bereavement books and grief experts that it's good to talk and good to cry. Of course, death does still come unexpectedly and tragically to the young and fit in all walks of life, through accidents, cancer and strokes, but these are *individual* disasters and experienced as personal tragedies. The number of occupational groups and geographical communities characterized by high rates of accidental death are now much reduced and along with them their *culture* of stoicism.

Tears: from human to feminine

Until the nineteenth century, grieving men were allowed to be as emotional as women. Vincent-Buffault (1991) traces how in eighteenth- and nineteenth-century France the rules and rhetoric of crying changed. Crying, once an open demonstration by both sexes, became more private, a sign of the feminine and the antithesis of the masculine. I have noted above how in the second third of the nineteenth century the public school ethos promoted the same shift in England. Grief came to be seen as particularly associated with women's frail, emotional nature. Tears moved from public demonstration to the privacy of the house. So mourning was carried out by women, in private, curtailing their social engagements and public appearances (Jalland 1996).

I have already noted how, in the first wave of feminism at the beginning of the twentieth century, educated women began to liberate themselves from the requirement to mourn. But without the Victorian etiquette of mourning, which carefully stipulated a time and a place (and a gender) for tears, how and when should tears be expressed? Women were left with few rules to follow, but they were still left with their tears. Is it coincidence that now, with the second wave of feminism and with women coming out of the private home and taking their place in the public realm – crucially, the realms of publishing, the broadcast media, and the personal growth movement – many are now at pains to state that there is no shame in the tears of grief (Simonds and Rothman 1992)? Suffice it to say here that the debate about the value of tears is a gendered debate and one with a gendered history (see Chapter 10).

From soul to corpse to psyche

When it comes to what is looked at after death, it is quite clear that, over time, there has been a shift in gaze. In the high Middle Ages, the living gazed at, prayed for and wondered about the state of the soul. Then in the early modern period, the gaze shifted toward the corpse. First, Renaissance humanists, whether doctors or artists, became interested in the dead body as an object to be studied. Second, Protestantism's reluctance to pray for the soul led to funerals that focused increasingly – in the eighteenth and nineteenth centuries – on the corpse, the coffin and the paraphernalia that went with the coffin. In addition, third, the failure of time-honoured burial practices to cope with the population pressures of the rapidly expanding cities of the nineteenth century caused a public health outcry. In the middle third of the century (50 years earlier in Paris), many European cities became preoccupied with reorganizing cemeteries so that the bodies of the dead did not adversely affect the physical health of the living. But by the last third of the century, as the high Victorian funeral declined and the burial crisis was solved by building large out-of-town cemeteries, so the gaze of the living shifted focus once more, this time to the psychological state of the bereaved.[5]

As we have seen, romanticism had been preoccupied with the feelings of loss ever since the graveyard poetry of the early eighteenth century and reached a high point in the mid-nineteenth. Once the corpse was removed as an object of concern, the gaze shifted to the mourners' emotions. At first, in the nineteenth century, the emotions of grief were clearly regulated. With the erosion of Victorian mourning, their regulation became altogether more problematic, the twentieth-century mourner (in England at any rate) becoming preoccupied with how to display the right level of grief when the rules were no longer so clear (see Chapter 8). By the last third of the twentieth century, bereavement literature positively celebrates the emotions of grief as good for psychological growth, with self-help manuals promoting healthy grief replacing etiquette books promoting respectable mourning. Most leaflets produced by bereavement organizations emphasize that all the emotions associated with grief are natural and healthy and any pathologizing or policing of them is unhelpful. Though the script has changed, the emotions of grief have nevertheless remained centre stage for over a century, with soul and corpse now consigned to the wings, barely visible.[6]

Comforters have also shifted their gaze, from scrutinizing the mourner's body to scrutinizing his or her emotions. In high Victorian mourning, as we see in Puckle's belated example of the house painter's widow, what mattered was whether she was wearing the right clothes for the right period of time and behaving in an appropriate manner. Mourning dress assured others that you were feeling the right things. But with mourning dress now abandoned, how will others know that you are grieving? They scrutinize you for the tell-tale but subtle signs of inner emotion, in order to know what you are really feeling and therefore how to relate to you. This is true of both popular culture (Chapter 8) and more formal bereavement care (Chapter 11).

Are mourning dress and social mourning staging a comeback? After the death of Princess Diana in 1997, tennis stars such as André Agassi and Greg Rusedski sported black ribbons – a variation on the red ribbons originally worn in solidarity for those with AIDS. You could tell who among the normal London crowds were mourners come to pay their tributes to Diana because they were clutching sprays of flowers. Whatever they actually felt, these insignia marked them out as bona fide mourners. On both sides of the Atlantic (Haney *et al.* 1997), flowers are now often left at the scene of road traffic accidents: so long as you have left your flowers, you have done your bit and no one can doubt that you have been touched by the death. In the UK, ritual remembrances for the war dead are on the increase. Some, however, heirs to a century of belief in authentically felt grief, are horrified at what appears to them as the beginnings of a reinstatement of socially required mourning.

Conclusion

This chapter has sketched some of the ways in which the emotions of grief have been regulated over the past four centuries. Sixteenth-century England promoted a cult of secular melancholy, fostered by a Puritanism that eschewed religious manifestations of grief. Adam Smith's theory of sympathy is then discussed, indicating its potential for a sociology of mourning. High Victorian mourning primarily concerned status and respectability, only to be rejected in the twentieth century by a private grief more in tune with personal feeling. There has also been a shift from spontaneous Victorian expressions of grief to a twentieth-century stoicism, born in part from two world wars; but with peace and affluence for much of the West in the second half of the century, a more expressive style is once again gaining ground. Simplifying this, we may say that the Middle Ages were concerned most with the deceased's soul, the Renaissance to the Enlightenment were fascinated by the corpse and the cemetery in which it lay, while the last two centuries have come increasingly to gaze upon the inner world of the bereaved survivor.

Further reading

Ariès, P. (1974) *Western Attitudes toward Death: From the Middle Ages to the Present*. Baltimore: Johns Hopkins University Press.

Morley, J. (1971) *Death, Heaven and the Victorians*. London: Studio Vista.

Taylor, L. (1983) *Mourning Dress: A Costume and Social History*. London: Allen & Unwin.

Questions

1 What are the rules of sympathy in the circles in which you mix?
2 When it comes to grief, would you want to be an upper-class Victorian woman?
3 Tears are a luxury of a peaceful, safe society. Discuss.

Notes

1 Goody and Poppi (1994: 153) observe that Italy embraces neither the northern European gothic lore of cemetery ghosts nor the modern horror movie.
2 Person-centred counsellors, however, may reveal thoughts or feelings that are a direct response to what the client has said or expressed (Mearns and Thorne 1988; McLaren 1998). This Rogerian notion of 'congruence' may not be so far removed from Smith's theory of condolence.
3 Sussex University, Mass Observation Archive.
4 James Ballard, Meet the Author, CRUSE/Bereavement Care annual conference, September 1997. See also Ballard (1996).
5 Elsewhere (Walter 1994; 1996a), I have documented how the shift of gaze from soul to body to psyche has in the West affected the period before death as well as the period after.
6 Elsewhere (Walter 1990), I have shown how this affects the contemporary funeral.

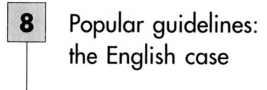

8 Popular guidelines: the English case

> Grief is like sex. It can be done on your own, is best done with one other, and is disapproved of if done in public.[1]

This chapter describes the popular guidelines for grief in the author's own culture, namely mainstream white English culture. By the 'English' I refer primarily to those of English descent, living in England, the *British* way of death being considerably more varied than the English.[2] White readers in Scotland, Wales, Australia, New Zealand and South Africa may find some similarities, as may some middle-class Protestant Northern Irish. Non-white readers in these countries may find it helpful to have dissected the mainstream culture of mourning with which they have to contend and may wish to identify those aspects of English mourning that they have absorbed and those they reject. North American readers may want to ask how much their own mourning culture shares with the English – I suspect the answer is quite a lot.

White English people are not prone to wearing their emotions on their sleeves and they are expected to bear suffering with a stiff upper lip. English men, in particular, are not supposed to weep and hug each other – except on the football field. Does this emotional reserve lead to a particular way of managing grief? In this chapter, I identify seven different social norms or scripts that govern the English way of grief. These scripts can conflict with one another and conflict can lead to change. Different members of the same family may hold different norms as to the proper way to grieve, causing rifts between members at a time when they most need to support each other. Awareness of, and respect for, these different scripts may help reduce this added isolation that bereaved people often face.

Table 8.1   Norms for grief (selected western societies)

	Formal (acceptance of ritual)	Informal (distrust of ritual)
Expressive	Ireland Mediterranean countries Orthodox Jews	Various parts of USA (e.g. West Coast)
Reserved	Scotland Germany Switzerland Finland	England Australia Netherlands Various parts of USA

Any study of grief in England has to refer to Geoffrey Gorer's much-cited *Death, Grief and Mourning in Contemporary Britain* (1965), based on a representative survey conducted in 1963. My other starting point is a short passage in *The Loneliness of the Dying* by Norbert Elias (1985). Elias argues that traditional rituals provided a framework within which you could express how you felt (pp.24–8), but nowadays we have become more informal (see also Wouters 1977, 1986) and distrust 'empty' ritual. This would not present problems for the mourner, were it not for the combination of informality with emotional reserve. Denied the old ritual forms in which strong emotion could be expressed in code, mourners now find that emotional reserve forbids any public expression of grief. But are informalization and emotional reserve inevitable in the development of western civilization (as Elias suggests) or do they characterize some nations more than others (as I will suggest)?

Using Elias's two dimensions of expressive/non-expressive and formal/informal, Table 8.1 shows how certain cultures vary on the two dimensions of expressiveness and formality, and thus how the English way of grief may differ from other modern western countries and indeed from other patterns within the British Isles.

Ireland, Italy, Greece and Orthodox Jews have clear funeral and mourning customs which ritualize emotion in a way that would embarrass most English. This is very different from the expressivism of parts of the USA, for example its West Coast, which distrusts ritual. Overall, the USA is a very informal and de-ritualized culture, but ranges over the whole spectrum from reserved to expressive. Cultures that *dis*courage public expression of the emotions of grief range from those that are rather formal in their rituals (Scotland, Germany, Switzerland and Finland) to those that are much more informal (England, Australia, Netherlands and various parts of the USA).[3] If Elias is correct that the combination of informality with reserve makes the articulation of grief particularly problematic, then this would apply to this last quartet.

Table 8.2 Norms for grief (British Isles)

	Formal (acceptance of ritual)	Informal (distrust of ritual)
Expressive	Irish (Catholic, working class) Orthodox Jewish Hindu Caribbean Muslim (female)	English (expressive professions) Diana, Princess of Wales
Reserved	English (traditional working class) Traditional Scottish Protestant Ulster (middle class) Royal Family Muslim (male)	English (commercial middle class, detraditionalized working class)

Table 8.2 relates the English way of grief to other patterns within the British Isles and identifies variations *within* the English way. This chapter refers mainly to the bottom right-hand box, consisting of the commercial section of the middle class and the detraditionalized members of the working class, comprising well over half the English population. Just as there are complexly intertwining norms within this group, so there are complexities and variations within all the other groups listed in Tables 8.1 and 8.2. The intention of this chapter is not to stereotype and pigeon-hole, say, Finns, Orthodox Jews or West Indians but to encourage readers from these communities to attempt the kind of analysis that I offer for my own community, namely to identify the conflicting and evolving ways in which grief is policed in their community. Wikan (1988), for example, observes that grieving Muslims in Egypt are expected to express their grief, while Muslims in Bali are expected to be cheerful and distract themselves; norms for grieving Muslims in Britain are doubtless as varied as those I describe in this chapter for my own community.

Personal grief

Gorer claimed that 'the style of mourning in Britain is now a matter of individual choice'. Until the beginning of this century all societies provided rules how to mourn (possibly, Gorer suggests, reflecting the preferred styles of powerful individuals), but in contemporary Britain 'the cultural rules are discarded (so) the varieties of individual temperament will develop spontaneously private behaviour' (Gorer 1965: 64). There is mounting evidence (Wortman and Silver 1989) that there is not one way through grief but several, so a norm of freedom could represent liberation from imposed rules of mourning. Certainly in my own experiences of loss from the early 1970s to the present, I have not felt any great social pressure to grieve in a certain way and I have been aware that others have grieved in different ways from myself.

When given total freedom, however, most human beings do not know how to use it, looking anxiously around to see how others are using theirs. In the 1830s de Tocqueville observed that Americans, a people who proclaim individual freedom as an absolute value, were actually rather conformist (Bellah *et al.* 1985). Throughout the modern West, teenagers loudly protest their freedom yet are desperate to make the same consumer choices as their peers. Bereavement is a stage of life evoking even more anxiety than adolescence, so even if there are no strong, nation-wide norms as to how to grieve, mourners still conform to certain patterns, often learnt within their nuclear family. Bereavement is a time of insecurity, the most unlikely moment for people to become pioneers or eccentrics, as any funeral director will tell you. Bereavement organizations often comment that their clients need to know that their emotions are normal and not signs that they are going mad; they are grateful to be informed that their emotions and responses are within the range of the normal.

Many contemporary books on grief, however, give examples of bereaved people being criticized for inappropriate behaviour, indicating that many of the English do not believe that mourning behaviour should be a matter of personal inclination. A widow with a young son and daughter said:

> I just couldn't cope for a long while, there was nothing to do for it. My sister and the minister told me to pull myself together, but I said 'What for?' They said I had to for the children, but I still felt there was nothing to do for it.
>
> (Marris 1958: 11)

In the previous chapter, we encountered Sir John Soane two centuries ago and Jeanne Blank in the USA today facing similar criticism. If indeed people do have their own preferred style of grieving, it can be very hard for other family members who have a different style. She wants to talk and talk and talk, he wants to go for long walks and visit the grave by himself. Couples who thought they knew each other begin to find the other behaving in incomprehensible ways, because of gender, personality or (Shapiro 1994; 1996) cultural differences that only grief brings to the fore. He remarries before his children have got over the loss of their mother. Gorer (1965: 81, 83) gives similar examples of criticism from grieving relatives and neighbours, and indeed he himself implicitly criticizes the style adopted by some of his interviewees.

Insofar as there is a norm of freedom to follow personal inclination, and there is, this does not mean the grieving are free from social influence. They may seek affirmation, or they may receive unasked for advice or criticism. Freedom does not exist in a social vacuum.

Anomic grief

Gorer concluded that for most Britons the abolition of culturally prescribed grieving did not result in personal freedom but in a de-regulation that left people at a loss. This is the state Durkheim termed anomie – though Gorer did not refer to Durkheim. The only exceptions, Gorer concluded, were the (then very small, but now somewhat larger) religious minorities that lay down clear rules and rituals for mourning.

Gorer argued that mid-twentieth century Britain had witnessed the demise of Victorian funeral and mourning rituals, leaving a vacuum. David Cannadine (1981) has challenged both Gorer's somewhat rosy view of Victorian mourning and his timing of its demise, but nevertheless affirms Gorer's identification of the importance of the First World War. After the carnage of the War, Cannadine argues, the peace-time death rate continued to decline, funerals became simpler, mourning less elaborate, yet there was a 'massive, all-pervasive pall of death which hung over Britain', and Cannadine writes of 'the inventiveness with which the grief-stricken responded to their bereavement.' (p.230) This inter-war period saw a flourishing of the cult of remembrance, pilgrimages to war graves and spiritualism.

Building on Cannadine's work, Ruth Richardson (1984) has suggested that each generation this century has had its own socialization into awareness of death. In the mid-1980s, many of the very old, raised before the First World War and some of them survivors of the trenches, had always known they were mortal – though the upper classes were protected as children from the sight of death. The generation raised between the wars seems to have grown up with a horror of morbid ritual, perhaps in reaction to the inter-war obsession with death, yet all too aware that some of their male relatives were missing – and were themselves in turn plunged into the Second World War. It is this generation, I suggest, that is most likely to be characterized now by anomie. It is certainly this generation that some of its children now castigate for 'denying' death. The post-1945 generation by contrast grew up under the abstract shadow of the bomb, but without direct contact with death – mortality rates were at an all-time low, most deaths occurred in hospital and children could grow up with the family still complete. Richardson (1984: 51) reckons this generation seems 'less worried by death than the shell-shocked generation born between the wars, children and grandchildren of the Great War's bereaved'.

If anomie is an accurate characterization of the grief of some Britons, we must be clear as to precisely which generation or generations are characterized by anomie. Clare Gittings[4] has observed that, whereas the late Middle

Ages and the seventeenth century saw the publication of many manuals on how to die but none on how to grieve, now the market is flooded with manuals on healthy grieving. Presumably the demand comes from people looking for guidance, as much from the post-war (now middle aged) as the inter-war (now elderly) generation. Arguably, several generations have experienced anomie, each in their different way. If norms for grieving arise in specific historical conditions and then get established, they are not easily abandoned even though circumstances change. At a time of grief, people are unlikely to want to change the rules. It may, therefore, be *normal* for grief to be policed according to rules that are no longer appropriate, leaving a proportion of people feeling that the rules do not work for them. Some of the mourner's confusion can derive from this, as well as from the grief itself.

Private grief

> The ladies of a bereaved family should not see callers, even intimate friends, unless they are able to control their grief. It is distressing alike to the visitor and the mourner to go through a scene of uncontrolled grief. Yet it is difficult to keep a firm hold over the emotions at such a time, and it is therefore wiser to see no one if there is a chance of breaking down ... Even relatives should remember that the bereaved ones will want to be by themselves, and that solitude is often the greatest solace for grief.
>
> (From an upper class etiquette book: Troubridge 1926: 57–8)

> No-one knows my sorrow
> Few have seen me weep
> I cry from a broken heart
> While others are asleep
>
> (Working class *In Memoriam* notice in
> regional newspaper, late 1970s)

The previous chapter documented how nineteenth-century socially required mourning evolved into the twentieth-century experience of private grief. The dominant norm in mid- to late twentieth-century Britain, starting with the upper classes and then filtering down the social ladder, is *private* grief. This clearly differentiates what is felt in private from what is shown in public, and is well understood by a people who value emotional reserve. The norm is that grief should be private and not disturb others; it should not go on indefinitely, for this too is disturbing to others. If these are the obligations of the grieving person, the obligation of others is not to intrude upon his or her grief. Gorer (1965: 113) captures this when he says of the British that 'one mourns in private as one undresses or relieves oneself in private, so as not to offend others.'[5] This can be problematic in institutions where private backstages are not so readily available. Carmichael (1991: ch.5) describes how in hospitals, staff cry not on the ward where their tears will upset the emotional order, but on the lavatory or in the office of the social worker or chaplain. Quite where bed-bound patients are supposed to cry is not stated.

The norm of private grief is even more problematic, however, than may at first sight appear. The norm is not just that you should grieve in private, but that others should *know* you are privately grieving – otherwise you might not have cared for your husband/mother/child after all! The *In Memoriam* notice quoted at the beginning of this section, published in the local newspaper, obeys this perfectly, letting everyone know how deeply the person feels, without a single public tear to cause embarrassment. The task for the grieving is to provide clues that they feel deeply, without actually breaking down in public. Those who cannot control their grief in public embarrass both themselves and others.

Such perfected control is, however, difficult to achieve. A relative reads the lesson at the funeral and momentarily has a catch in his voice but masters this and continues to read the lesson perfectly; a funeral attender dabs at a moist eye but does not break down; the widow answers a telephone call of condolence with the occasional halt in her voice but continues to appreciate or even enjoy the conversation – all these have mastered the fine art of English grief. Breaking down in the privacy of your own room is to be expected, though – as Marris's (1958) study of younger widows in the 1950s makes very clear – not in front of the children. This difficulty of pulling off a successful performance could explain why friends and neighbours may avoid mourners, or mourners avoid their friends and neighbours.

The norm that grief should be private makes any public appearance problematic, and the emotionally charged appearance at the funeral particularly so. After the funeral, mourners say of the widow on view to all in the front row of the crematorium 'Didn't she do well?' – signifying a successful performance in which she did not break down but gave off enough signals to indicate she was feeling terrible. Though they may look back on the funeral as a success – a 'great occasion' or a 'wonderful tribute' to the dead person – that is not the attitude with which they entered the funeral. They anticipate it to be a trial of emotional strength and acting skill to be got over and done with as soon as possible. People who normally avoid mood-altering medication will take valium for this one occasion.

According to stage theories of grief, the funeral tends to occur during the first, numb, stage – which experts who want the funeral to be therapeutic may deem to be bad timing. Or they may hope that the stark reality of the funeral will de-freeze the numbness – which on a number of occasions it indeed does. But many people *prefer* to be numb at the funeral as this reduces the chances of their causing a scene; some may subconsciously choose to keep the numbness going until the funeral. (Mediterranean and West Indian funerals can occur soon after the death, but are not noted for emotional numbness.)

Managing the appearance of a privately grieving self is particularly tricky now that Victorian ritual mourning is no more. Victorian mourning clothes, particularly the middle- or upper-class widow's black dress and veil, hid how she really felt, as did her enforced absence from social engagements. In the twentieth century, the display of grief has to be consciously staged by the individual. Widows and widowers must display that they are upset in more subtle ways, such as the temporarily broken voice or the careful timing and management of meetings with potential future partners.

The desire not to break down in front of the children is well documented, in North America (Silverman 1986: 94–6; Prince 1996) as well as in Britain (Carmichael 1991: ch.6). This may derive from a desire to protect children from intense pain, or from a belief that children are not able to experience grief. Or it may derive from precisely the opposite; it may be the very openness and naïvety of grieving children that cause the parent to withdraw – one such American widow compared her children's questions to 'a knife being stuck in my throat' (Silverman 1986: 93). But if parents' grief is private, how are children to learn about grief? If all that can be observed in public is the stiff upper lip, how will first-time mourners know what is 'normal'? How will they know whether their feelings are 'normal'? How will they know when they should be 'getting over it'? The answer often is that they do not, which could be one reason for the contemporary demand for grief manuals and the reassurance offered in counselling as to what is normal grief. It could also be a reason for the growth of autobiographical accounts of loss (Holloway 1990) and of personal revelations in bereavement groups where mourners share their feelings and experiences with each other. The mass media, especially soap operas and the news, also provide role models for mourning (Walter et al. 1995).

The dual process model (Stroebe and Schut 1999) provides a psychological interpretation of private grief. Private grief entails oscillating between feeling the pain (at home, behind closed doors) and getting on with life (in public). This is precisely the oscillation that Stroebe and Schut speak of, namely that bereaved people have to move back and forth between emotion-focused grief work and task-focused learning of new roles and skills. Stroebe and Shut observe that the two cannot be done at the same time, which is precisely what private grief assumes: there is no need for the stiff upper lip when you are grieving at home, and it is unwise to let grief invade the execution of your public roles at work and with friends.

As noted in Table 8.2, the Irish ritualize their grief in a much more expressive and public manner. This English/Irish difference can lead to difficulties for those who must cross the divide. A 30-year-old Irish woman, who had grown up in England but went back to the West Coast of Ireland for her father's funeral, was disturbed by being expected to weep with up to 200 villagers whom she had never met before. She much preferred the more private English way of grief. Prior (1989: 141–52) shows that in Northern Ireland, both class and religion affect notions of privacy in grief, so that middle-class Protestants are closest to the English reserve, while Catholics and working-class people routinely engage in extensive public declarations of grief and of sympathy. Inviting television cameras to film terrorist funerals may seem the depth of bad taste to English viewers but is simply normal in a working-class Irish culture where funerals are dramatic public affairs for the whole community, and the bigger the congregation the better.

Forbidden grief

Forbidden grief occurs when others deny the person has suffered any loss. Losing a partner in a covert homosexual relationship is one example, losing a mistress or lover can be another. Miscarriage and stillbirths were also once in this category – 'just one of those things' that parents must put behind them. This, however, has been challenged in the past decade. Whereas previously a stillbirth would not have received any ritual or personal attention, many maternity units now encourage parents to hold their dead baby and attend its funeral, while books are now published on the psychological trauma of miscarriage.

Very common, as we shall see below in the section on time-limited grief, is when friends and family want the (usually female) mourner to put her grief behind her sooner than she wants. With loss of a child, the parent may object to the idea that she should ever 'get over it'. In such instances, we have private grief followed by forbidden grief.

Time-limited grief

Gorer argued that healthy grieving is time limited – neither forbidden, nor prolonged indefinitely. He suggested that time-limited grieving characterizes many traditional cultures, but that not all of the Britons he interviewed managed it. I would argue that, though many English people grieve a shorter time than Gorer thought healthy, the idea that grief should last only a certain amount of time is very common. The idea is that you should get back to normal, especially emotional normality, as soon as possible. This is often implied in criticism:

> My family were very nice for about six weeks – very understanding but I was terrible for months afterwards, I used to forget things – I was living in another world, it takes me a long time to get over things. Anyway in the end they just lost patience. My husband was really

nasty about it, he said: 'For God's sake woman what's the matter with you, I was never like that when my mother died – it's been *months*.'
(Littlewood 1992: 87)

The trouble is partly that nobody can agree what 'as soon as possible' means. Littlewood points out that the decline of socially imposed mourning means that mourners now have to negotiate their own time limits; this can only be done with their significant others, and there may not be agreement, as in the above quote. While many bereaved people value the support given, after a time, to re-engage in social activities or to take up paid work, 40 per cent of those interviewed by Littlewood felt the withdrawal of emotional support was premature. Employers often expect you to be back to normal in a matter of days.

The difficulties of agreeing, when etiquette is no longer written in books, when an end to mourning is appropriate became news both after the Hillsborough disaster of 1989 and after the death of Diana, Princess of Wales in 1997. There was considerable discussion in the national press about when it would be appropriate for certain key football matches to be played after their postponement in the days immediately following Hillsborough (Walter 1991b). Around eight months after her death, there was public debate as to if and when the Diana memorial fund should cease to accept donations, and both Diana's brother, Earl Spencer, and Elton John (who sang at her funeral) pleaded that the media cease its obsessive coverage of the death and let them, and the world, get on with life.

Distracted grief

Among the Victorian upper classes, mourning women were expected to stay at home and indulge their grief, but mourning men were advised to distract themselves by returning to work as soon as possible. Caroline Fox wrote of one widower, after his wife's sudden death in 1838, 'What will become of poor Lord John? His plunging into business at once is his best chance of struggling against the sadness'. Likewise, Sir Warwick Morshead's response to his wife's death was to 'throw myself into everything that I can, which distracts thought, and now I am busy about setting up a workman's club in the village' (Jalland 1996: 252).

Distracting yourself is advice frequently given to mourners of both sexes and all classes in the late twentieth century. According to reminder theory (Rosenblatt *et al.* 1976) and oscillation theory (Stroebe and Schut 1999), it is particularly good advice, especially for housewives who may need distractions from a home that continually reminds them of the dead husband or child. (The requirement that upper-class Victorian widows shut themselves up at home for a year may have been particularly bad advice, unless the intention was to show them how terrible life was without a man.)

Silverman's study of American widows (1986: ch.9) and Riches and Dawson's study of British bereaved parents (1997) both found different styles of grieving according to the roles and identities embraced by the mourners. Widows who went out to work found this distracted them, they tended to avoid their feelings, and on the whole they seemed to cope better than those who were engulfed by their grief. Some widows have reported that getting a job was the best thing they ever did. Likewise, those bereaved parents (female as well as male) who found meaning in work as well as in parenthood were able to find distractions from grief and support from those outside the home.

Expressive grief

Collick (1986) describes a meeting of 40 widows and widowers discussing their spouse's funerals:

> Some aware of themselves as the centre of interest, felt called upon to act a part that did not fit with their genuine feelings:
> 'I wasn't thinking of myself at all, mostly wondering who was there and what they would be feeling.'
> 'It's the one day you don't care or feel for yourself. You keep going for others.'
> Some wanted to cry and could not; others cried and felt they should not:
> 'Shoulders back, head up, mustn't let the side down.'
> 'I had to behave well for his sake.'
> It seemed that most felt behaviour was what mattered.
>
> (Collick 1986: 25)

Collick describes well the difficulty of keeping grief private in the public situation of the funeral. She also provides evidence for Adam Smith's theory of condolence: the widows and widowers hold back on public displays of grief in an attempt to match that of the other mourners (whose grief may have been heightened by the funeral). The funeral is an occasion which each person attends for the sake of others: the mourners attend in order to support the widow, the widow attends because the funeral is the only occasion other mourners will have to say farewell to the deceased; they are all there out of respect for the dead. The funeral for these widows and widowers is primarily a social performance, conducted for the sake of others.

Yet Collick's interpretation ignores all this and implies that the funeral ought to be an occasion for the expression of personal grief. Though the widows and widowers themselves do not, Collick contrasts 'acting a part' with 'their genuine feelings', and she is unsympathetic with their feeling that behaviour was important for the sake of their deceased spouses and for the sake of the other mourners. On the previous page she had asserted that 'a funeral . . . gives the bereaved permission to grieve', despite the clear evidence to the contrary from her widows and widowers. What she presumably means is that funerals *ought* to allow the bereaved to grieve, but at present typically do not. Collick is an advocate of a movement that is currently promoting the idea that mourning should express inner feeling not social expectation.

Over the past two to three decades, private grief has been severely criticized by those who consider it psychologically healthy for people to be more expressive. For expressivists, 'the grief process' entails 'working through' and/or expressing a range of feelings – a view often propagated by what Bernice Martin (1981) terms Britain's expressive professions (clergy, social workers, nurses, teachers, etc). Gorer himself is an expressivist, but the most influential expressivist has been the Swiss American Elisabeth Kübler-Ross (1970) whose best selling text on the stages of dying was taken to describe stages of grief as well. The expressivist revolution in death and dying has been described in some detail by sociologists Lofland (1978), Wood (1977) and Walter (1994). The intellectual origin of the revolution is the Freudian idea of repression; the social origin is the strand in American culture that Bellah *et al.* (1985) term expressive individualism; and the immediate historical origin is the counter-culture of the 1960s. The vast majority of the current books and media documentaries on bereavement are produced by expressivists aiming to challenge private, personal and anomic grief. There is one healthy way to grieve, they believe, and – having got the media on their side – are making sure we all know what it is.

That the British have not immediately taken to expressing grief, indeed to a considerable extent reject it, is in part because – unlike private grief – expressive grief takes little or no account of the distinction between public and private. Expressivists see emotion as contained within the human body, waiting to erupt like pressure from a steam engine, rather than – as in many cultures – a scripted performance, with understood rules (Sarbin 1986a; Hockey 1993). Expressivists see the expression of grief not as social but as natural; it is therefore harmful to repress tears – whatever the situation. Public situations, however, are not natural but are governed by social rules. Expressive grief also leaves the bereaved person totally dependent on the goodwill of others, while private grief and Adam Smith's theory of condolence both allow a degree of reciprocity: the bereaved are expected to adjust their behaviour to assist their would-be comforters, as well as vice-versa, and their comforters appreciate the effort.

All this cannot but leave millions of Britons confused. They are now encouraged to cry, yet are aware that encounters with others are rule-governed and that weeping spontaneously in supermarket, hospital ward or outside the school gates will disturb. Expressivists provide no guidance as to when, how, in what manner or with which people it is appropriate to express grief. In many ways the old norm, that you grieve alone while holding yourself together in public, is much easier. For the new norm to take hold, the emphasis on tears as psychologically healthy must be complemented by guidelines as to when and where is the best place to cry. Otherwise the anxiety level of people who are bereaved, not to mention everybody else, cannot but rise. This is so in any western society, but especially so in a society that values emotional reserve – which is why expressivist literature emanating from a less reserved California may not be totally helpful to grieving English men and women, or for that matter New Englanders. The new norm may therefore develop into but a variation of the old – grieve in private (private being extended to include one-to-one encounters with a trusted friend or counsellor) but not in public.

Another area where expressivism comes into direct conflict with the norm of emotional reserve is at the funeral. Increasingly textbooks refer to the funeral as an occasion for expressing emotion, yet mourners – and clergy (Hockey 1993) – are often petrified of uncontrollable emotion in funerals. There is in fact no widespread demand for more emotional funerals. Funerals must affirm the mourners' cultural values in order to stabilize their fragile grasp on reality, so the English are unlikely to approve of funerals that challenge emotional reserve. Indeed, the English often criticize Irish funerals for being 'sentimental' or 'wild'. What *is* widely wanted in England, however, is for funerals to be more personal. The English seem to like funerals that capture the personality of the deceased and criticize those that do not (Walter 1990).

In the wake of the revolution described in Chapter 6, there are now a number of publications challenging expressivism, making assertions that everybody grieves differently, which are neatly summarized in Ironside's (1996: xvii) observation that 'You do not work through bereavement. It works through you.' These publications are promoting my first type, personal grief. But these critics are vulnerable to the weakness of personal grief: it can easily collapse into anomie, with people wanting assurance that their grief is appropriate.

Death of a princess

What, then, about Princess Diana's funeral? Did this, as press and commentators alleged, mark a radical shift toward a more expressive Englishness?[6] Basically, no, and for two reasons (Biddle and Walter 1998; Walter 1999b). First, the impression of a nation in tears was largely generated by media camera operators and editors who, for reasons of their own, were on the lookout for emotion. Of the mourners standing in line to sign a book of condolence, the one in tears made a better photograph than the 99 in sombre silence. The press had in any case for some years been interested in the phenomenon of 'the emotional male', highlighting the tears of macho footballers on missing the crucial penalty shot, and the crowds that gathered to mourn Princess Diana provided enough material of this kind to develop this particular story. But the overall impression of those present was of a respectful silence, a very English standing in line, with sobs noticeable primarily because they punctuated the overwhelming silence.

Second, insofar as tears were shed for Diana, and many certainly were, this did not mark any major change in how more ordinary deaths have been subsequently grieved. (Diana's funeral *has* furthered the already existing trend toward more personal funerals, but as I have just said above, more personal funerals are not necessarily more emotional.) What happened after Diana's death was a national, to some extent global, reversion to a traditional mourning pattern in which a whole community is required to mourn the death of a high profile member, with the added dimension of shock at the unexpected death of one who seemed so vibrant and invincible. Widespread, and to an extent emotional, mourning in such circumstances is not so unexpected; it is a product of specific circumstances. Strangers who hugged each other in Hyde Park on the day of the funeral were as private as ever the next time someone more ordinary, or someone more personally known, died.

The mourning for Diana does, however, suggest that support for expressivism may be spreading beyond Martin's expressive professions. Diana was herself an ambassador for expressiveness – which put the informal, expressive princess in direct conflict with the formal, reserved Windsors (Table 8.2). That her informal expressiveness, her conviction that you solve your problems by talking about them (to therapists or to the world) not by hiding them, drew support from millions of people (mainly 20–40-year-old lower-middle and upper-working class females) who had hitherto been sceptical of social workers and therapists. This may indicate a wider base of support for expressiveness than I had hitherto thought, but professional counsellors tell me it has yet to show in attitudes toward bereavement.

Practical implications

Just as it is misleading to think that each ethnic minority in the UK has its own unitary and coherent way of grief (Gunaratnam 1997), so too the white English are subject to complex, contradictory and changing norms. This can cause difficulties for grieving people when two or more people mourn the same person but in different ways, or when mourner and comforter have different ideas of the proper way to grieve. Bereavement workers should be on the lookout for such problems, and they should also be aware of their own norms, where they fit on the cultural map and whether their norms have any more universal validity than anyone else's. This is particularly, and frequently, an issue for workers trained according to the expressive norm who face clients who embrace private grief.

Esther Shapiro (1994, 1996), writing from an American context strongly influenced by immigration and inter-ethnic marriage, has a helpful suggestion here. She works from the assumption that people grieve in varied ways, but the way that feels right to any particular individual may not gain support from the cultural expectations and required rituals of their family or community. The aim of therapy, according to Shapiro, is to help the client explore the goodness of fit between personal style and group expectation. A person's culture of origin, submerged for years of living in America or after years of marriage to someone from another culture, may resurface in ways of coping with stressful events such as bereavement, much to the surprise of spouse or children. This is particularly likely if the deceased had a symbolic significance in the drama of immigration: the parent who immigrated to the States, the child for whose all-American education so much was sacrificed. Shapiro's therapeutic model of identifying the fit between personal grieving style and cultural expectation could be easily adapted to the British context.

Summary

This chapter argues that the scripts for grief available in a society depend, in part, on whether the society values formality or informality, and whether it values expressiveness or reserve. England, tending toward informality and reserve, is taken as a case study. At least seven different scripts, or norms, can be identified: personal grief, anomic grief, private grief, forbidden grief, time-limited grief, distracted grief and expressive grief. Private grief is the dominant English script, but bereavement workers often advocate a more expressive script.

Further reading

Gorer, G. (1965) *Death, Grief, and Mourning in Contemporary Britain.* London, Cresset.
Shapiro, E. (1996) Family bereavement and cultural diversity: a social developmental model. *Family Process*, 35(4): 313–32.

Questions

1 What expectations – if any – have you experienced as to how you should grieve? Have these fitted or conflicted with how you yourself wanted to grieve?

2 What different expectations about healthy or proper grief are there in your own family?

3 What did you learn about grief as a child through observing others?

4 Create a role play based on Shapiro's therapeutic model.

Notes

1 Colin Murray Parkes, Mind and Mortality conference, London 19 March 1997.

2 *Great Britain* consists of England, Wales and Scotland; *the United Kingdom* consists of Great Britain plus Northern Ireland. *The British* are the citizens of the United Kingdom. *The British Isles* consist of Great Britain, Ireland and nearby smaller islands. *The Irish* are those from both Northern Ireland and the Republic of Ireland.

3 Outsiders see England as embracing ritual – the Monarchy, Beefeaters at the Tower of London, the Church of England, etc. But English culture generally is informal, certainly contrasted to German and Swiss.

4 Conference at St Alfred's College, Winchester, November 1996.

5 Elias (1978) suggests that the hiding of such bodily functions is typical of the civilizing process, but I suggest that its extension to grief characterizes some nations more than others.

6 Though Diana was, of course, mourned in Wales and Scotland, this was more marked in England.

9 Expert guidelines: clinical lore

It is often necessary to confront the patient gently but firmly with the reality of his situation, and to force him into a period of depression while he works out his acceptance of his loss.

(Nemiah 1957: 146)

There are three main stages of grief that everyone must pass through ... Everyone has to go through the stages of grief so that they can accept the reality of loss, bear the pain, adjust to a world in which the dead person is missing and re-invest emotional energy in their new life. Failure to go through these processes leads to protracted grief and psychological and physical illness. Family, friends, doctors and counsellors need to act as supports and guides for the bereaved, helping them through the various stages.

(Porter 1996)

There is no prescription for how to grieve properly for a lost spouse, and no research-validated guideposts for what is normal vs deviant mourning ... We are just beginning to realize the full range of what may be considered 'normal' grieving.

(Zisook and Shuchter 1986: 288)

Defining clinical lore

In the last chapter I looked at popular culture and its expectations as to how people should grieve. Throughout the book I have referred to research studies into bereavement. Both popular culture and the research community have their own 'knowledge' about bereavement, but between the two exists an intermediary level, which, following Wortman and Silver (1989), I term 'clinical lore'. Clinical lore is the received wisdom that informs the work of more or less trained pratitioners who work in either a paid or a voluntary capacity with bereaved people; it includes the ways in which bereavement workers are trained, along with books and articles on bereavement intended for the general public. Clinical lore is much more important than research knowledge in the policing of bereaved individuals, for clinical lore is effectively the filter through which research knowledge reaches and controls the public.

That said, it is not always easy distinguishing clinical lore from research. Organizations such as the (North American) Association for Death Education and Counseling, while primarily consisting of practitioners in counselling and education, also include leading researchers. Many members of the (British) Bereavement Research Forum are practitioners. Many researchers have their own clinical practice; many practitioners do research. The British magazine *Bereavement Care* is intended for counsellors but includes up-to-date research reports. Nor is the distinction between clinical lore and popular culture always so distinct. Cruse, the UK's biggest bereavement care organization, has until recently given its volunteers only 40 hours basic training, and my impression is that for many of them the counselling they conduct is informed mainly by their own experience of bereavement and by their intuitive understanding of how to relate to another human being in distress; they sit pretty lightly to the theoretical models with which they were presented in training. Despite these difficulties of distinguishing what precisely constitutes clinical lore, I believe it is a useful concept for understanding how bereavement in the contemporary West is policed and patrolled.

Should the knowledge generated by mutual-help groups be counted as part of clinical lore? (I refer here to self-run groups, not those set up by counselling organizations.) On the one hand these groups typically reject popular culture with its notion of getting over grief in a matter of weeks, but on the other hand they typically also reject clinical lore with its notions of resolution, stages and normality. One could even go so far as to say it is precisely their rejection of these two bodies of knowledge that members actually use to define their group as distinct. The knowledge of self-help groups is probably best considered as a fourth kind of knowledge about bereavement, sometimes fitting in with, sometimes conflicting with, both clinical lore and research findings, and almost always conflicting with popular culture.

One might expect that bereavement workers would be very open to the uniqueness of each individual client and be reluctant to make generalizations about bereavement – and indeed there are practitioners like that (primarily counsellors trained according to the person-centred school). By the same token, one might expect academic researchers, whose calling is to identify patterns in the infinite complexity of human behaviour, to be willing to make generalizations about bereavement – and indeed there are some researchers like that. In practice, however, things are often not like this. We find that practitioners often generalize about bereavement, referring for example to 'the grief process' as though there is just one way to grieve. We find that researchers typically hedge their conclusions with caveats, remind us how much data still needs to be collected before theories can be propounded with any degree of certainty, and in the meantime are very aware how many people do not fit their theories. In other words, those called to identify patterns hesitate to state what these patterns are, while those called to respecting individuality often generalize wildly!

The elements of clinical lore

Clinical lore in the early 1990s had the following main elements. First, expressivism. Mourners must confront and speak of their personal feelings, and if they do not they will suffer either physically or psychologically. As we have seen, this brings clinical lore into a head-on clash with much of the popular wisdom about grief, though aligns it with the expressive professions and their patron saint, Diana, Princess of Wales.

Second, grief should not go on for too long, and grief should sooner or later be 'resolved'. After a year or so, the mourner should have begun in significant ways to let go of the deceased and return to emotional stability. Letting go is in line with popular prescriptions though not (Part One) with the actual experience of all bereaved people, while the return to emotional stability is in line with both popular prescription and personal experience. The prescription that grief be time-limited fits popular culture conceptually, but expands the specified period radically from a month or two to a year or two; it conflicts conceptually with the experience of many people that grief has no end.

Third, clinical lore ties these ideas up in the notion of normal grief (i.e. expressing your feelings, letting go and returning to emotional normality after a year or two) and abnormal grief (not expressing your feelings, not letting go, still in a mess years later).

Jalland (1996: 12) found that the material written by and for upper-class Victorian mourners offered four primary sources of consolation: first and foremost, a religious belief in a happy family reunion, followed by the healing power of time, private and shared memory, and the sympathy of friends and relatives. A study of late twentieth-century literature on maternal grief found three very different kinds of comfort to be prominent: stories of other people's loss, information about the stages of grief, and affirmation that the emotions of grief are normal (Simonds and Rothman 1992: 158). This is reflected in contemporary books for other kinds of grief. Whereas Victorian comfort linked you physically to the living and spiritually to the dead, contemporary clinical lore, while symbolically linking you to an imagined community of grievers (Seale 1998), primarily informs you about your own psychological responses.[1]

It must be stated that professional counsellors trained according to the person-centred school of thought (Mearns and Thorne 1988) reject much of clinical lore (McLaren 1998). One such counsellor wrote to me about her practice:

> I resist your stating that professional counselling has notions of resolution, stages and normality as an integral part of its functioning. Some of us do not have notions of resolution, stages or even normality: we try to accept each bereaved client with whatever that person brings us by way of thoughts, feelings and behaviours. The whole notion of pathological grief is one which I find alien.

It is not known what proportion of bereavement workers operate in this way and what proportion operate according to clinical lore. There is rather little writing from a person-centred perspective specifically on bereavement and this can be misleading: bereavement care may actually be more diverse than the dominant themes in bereavement literature lead one to suppose.

Normality versus diversity

As described in Chapter 6, clinical lore is currently facing a revolution in which holding on to the deceased and a diversity of ways through grief are acknowledged. However, the three elements – expressivism, resolution, and some notion of normal and abnormal grief – are remarkably resilient, even in writings that otherwise seem to accept diversity. Defending this position, Colin Murray Parkes (personal communication) argues that

> The observation that everybody grieves differently is not incompatible with the idea that some ways of grieving give rise to more problems than others. It is a weakness that anthropological studies seldom attempt to measure differences in psycho-social adjustment between cultures, and tend to assume that whatever is culturally 'normal' is psychologically healthy.

In this view, diversity is acknowledged, but the concept of psychological pathology/abnormality is retained.

Thus, even when clinical lore does admit that there are many different ways of grieving, it typically at the same time tells us that the expressive way is best. Introductory leaflets by bereavement agencies illustrate this well, usually giving contradictory messages. One is that there is no right way to grieve and the other is that expressing emotion is the right way. For example, 'DO accept that people grieve in different ways. Allow them to let their feelings "out", rather than keep them "in"' (A Journey Through Bereavement, North West Hospice, 1996). Clinical lore does not simply say that everyone grieves differently; it makes authoritative claims about what is and is not healthy grieving.

Some bereavement workers may welcome this because it provides clear guidelines, rather than simply saying that everyone grieves differently. The publisher's catalogue advertising two books on working with grieving children, for example, cites reviews from practitioners' journals that praise them for mapping the typical ways in which children grieve, until recently somewhat uncharted territory. The books are, significantly, subtitled, 'The Forgotten Mourners: *Guidelines* for working with bereaved children' and 'Grief in Children: A *handbook* for adults' (my emphases), and the cited reviews include:

> 'gives clear and concise guidance on how children grieve . . . a useful and easy read . . . I particularly like the outlines for the process of grieving for different age groups . . .'

> 'offers an easy to follow introduction to supporting bereaved children.'
> (Pennells and Smith 1994)

> 'Dyregrov's writing is clear in its description, and explicit in its advice, and demonstrates that the daunting task of helping a child through grief is both manageable and rewarding.'
> (Dyregrov 1991)

The second of the Pennells and Smith reviews is from a newsletter for parents, indicating that they as well as practitioners may value guidance as to what is normal.

The primacy of feelings

The late Susan le Poidevin, a respected trainer of bereavement workers in the UK, observed that bereavement can affect people's identity, emotions, the spiritual meaning they give to life, the managing of practical everyday tasks, their physical health, their finances, their lifestyle (e.g. moving house, starting work) and their roles in family and community. Le Poidevin suggested that the practitioner should be aware of these many possible areas of distress and difficulty, and pick up on whichever are manifested by any particular client. This is very much in line with person-centred counselling, but goes against the direction in which bereavement care has been evolving in the second half of the twentieth century, namely away from practical help with a range of tasks and toward a preoccupation with the emotions of grief (Torrie 1987).

The multi-dimensional approach sits in tension with the dominant idea in clinical lore and in bereavement training, namely that just one dimension – the emotional – is what grief is *really* all about. William Worden's textbook (1983/1992), one of the most widely used in the English speaking world, identifies four tasks that bereaved people must accomplish: (1) accept the reality of the loss, (2) experience the pain of grief, (3) adjust to an environment without the deceased, and (4) withdraw emotionally from (first edition, 1983) / relocate (second edition, 1992) the deceased and move on with life. Worden's roots in Freud are obvious: the pain of life without the beloved has to be felt if heart as well as head is to come to terms with it and energy redirected into living once again.

A respected textbook titled *Gift of Tears: A Practical Approach to Loss and Bereavement Counselling* has a chapter on 'Basic Loss Counselling Skills', which includes exercises for the would-be bereavement worker. One is an exercise in listening skills:

> Restate in different words, and in clear and simple language, the literal meaning of the client's statements. Example:
> *Susan: My husband was a fine man. His sudden death was a great shock. I still miss him terribly.*
> One of the many possible responses from the counsellor might be:
> *Counsellor: Your husband's unexpected death really shook you to the core. You still miss him terribly.*
> (Lendrum and Syme 1992: 89)

This exercise encourages the student to translate any ostensibly objective statements about the deceased into statements about what the bereaved subjectively feels. The first sentence, 'My husband was a fine man', is ignored, perhaps because it is not so easily translated. Susan's cue that she wants to talk about her husband, which in person-centred counselling would be picked up, is simply dropped. Her second sentence, 'His sudden death was a great shock', could have meant that it was a great shock to many people; the husband could have been a headteacher who collapsed of a heart attack during school assembly, but it is translated simply into what it felt like for her. The final sentence, 'I still miss him terribly' is translated verbatim, as it already is in subjective format. The real give-away is that the exercise privileges this restatement into the language of feelings as the 'literal' meaning of what the client is saying. Statements about the deceased are thus superficial. Feelings, not statements about the deceased, constitute the discourse of grief counselling, at least according to this exercise.

Hockey (1986), an anthropologist who trained as a Cruse volunteer, confirms that this is precisely what Cruse training required her to do. Although active listening, practised in a wide variety of settings, is supposed simply to reflect back what the client has said, in bereavement work it typically *translates* what has been said into the language of feelings. In my own experience as a client of therapy, it is precisely the therapist's translation of what I have said that I have found helpful (or unhelpful). In much bereavement training, however, the translation has to be into one particular language – the language of feelings, rather than, say, the language of meaning, a major discourse of palliative and especially of spiritual care (Frankl

1964; Saunders 1988), or the language of physical ailments, a major discourse of general practitioners.

In addition to being helped to discover, articulate and ventilate painful feelings, clients (according to clinical lore) often find it helpful to be told that their feelings are normal and that they are not going mad. Clinical lore does not, however, see anger, blame and guilt to refer in any realistic way to the actual causes of the death, but to psychological realities within the mourner, which have to be suffered in order to arrive at inner healing. The cause of these feelings is 'the grief process', not the negligence of a car driver, a surgeon or the survivor, let alone the racism, poverty and social inequality that underlie so many deaths (Simonds and Rothman 1992: 164–72).

Insofar as bereavement care does acknowledge external causes for such emotions, it rarely gets involved in political or legal campaigning, concentrating instead on helping the client deal with these difficult emotions. This is one reason why politically active mutual help groups typically part company with more conventional bereavement organizations, developing instead the opposite (and equally extreme) ideology: that anger derives *entirely* from external factors and has nothing to do with grief. Such groups are pervaded by a culture of anger that positively drives members into campaigning action, but puts off some newcomers who perceive the anger to be an over-reaction (Rock 1998).

Grief work

Clinical lore is heavily committed to the idea of 'grief work', the hard work of experiencing the pain of loss, which is necessary if the person is to let go and move on.[2] This has been the principle underlying several specific programmes, which Stroebe (1992–3: 23) itemizes: 'regrief therapy' (Volkan), 'flooding' the client with pain-evoking stimuli (Ramsay) or gradually producing exposure to such stimuli (Gauthier and Pye), 'forced mourning' (Lieberman), 'reliving, revisiting and reviewing' (Melges and DeMaso), and so on. You get the idea from the first two quotes at the start of this chapter.

Whether grief work is actually necessary, however, has recently become a matter for debate. Stroebe has reviewed the evidence and concludes that 'Not only is there very little scientific evidence on the grief work hypothesis, but studies that bear on the issue yield contradictory results' (1992–3: 23, see also Pennebaker *et al.* forthcoming). Wortman and Silver's review of the research literature (1989) discovers that a number of those who do grief work have poorer, rather than better, outcomes. Stroebe *et al*'.s (1994) critique of Wortman and Silver suggests that they are referring here to those who engage in unconstructive and depressive rumination rather than emotionally cathartic grief work, yet agree that there is little positive evidence that active grief work is essential – although it can help widowers, it seems to have no benefit for widows. More recently, the research of Bonanno (forthcoming) and his colleagues at the Catholic University of America throws doubt on the conventional wisdom in clinical lore that the more openly people express negative thoughts and feelings in the earlier stages of bereavement, the sooner they will recover. Usually, genuine laughter, smiling and positive thoughts are correlated with shorter and less severe grief. Bonanno's research fits the arguments of Rosenblatt *et al.* (1976) and Stroebe and Schut (1999) that some distancing from unpleasant emotion is needed. It also fits the power of positive thinking, a popular idea in North America for several decades.

Why has clinical lore embraced the necessity for grief work?[3] The popularity of Worden's (1983/1991) book on helping the bereaved complete four 'tasks' may shed some light. Bereaved people, especially bereaved parents and those who have endured a sudden and unexpected loss, often find life unbearable because it is out of control. The trouble for them with 'stage' or 'phase' models of grief is that there is not much they can do but grieve and passively wait for the next stage to descend on them. The idea of working through tasks, however, gives the bereaved something to do; in returning to them some control over their lives, they are put back in touch with their former view of both themselves and of an orderly universe. The less fatalistic and the more activist the culture to which they belong, the more important this is likely to be – hence perhaps the popularity of 'grief work' in the USA.

Stages and schedules

A number of influential texts on bereavement identify phases that bereaved people typically go through or work through.

> Numbness, the first stage, gives place to pining, and pining to disorganization and despair, and it is only after the stage of disorganization that recovery occurs ... There are considerable differences from one person to another as regards both the duration and the form of each stage. Nevertheless there is a common pattern whose features can be observed without difficulty in nearly every case, and this justifies our regarding grief as a distinct psychological process.
>
> (Parkes 1986: 27)

Like Elizabeth Kübler-Ross with her famous five stages of dying (1970), these authors take great care to point out that these phases rarely occur in a straight, linear fashion. Rather waves, or pangs, of grief can resurface at any time, though this is likely to recur less and less often over time.

Unfortunately, and these authors are very aware of this, there are many people out there, not least the anxious young medical and nursing students who have to learn about grief but have not themselves lost anybody close, who want to be given simple and clear information about bereavement. They remember the neat pattern of stages and phases, and forget the caveats about it not being a simple linear process. Bereaved people themselves may also want a clear map of where they are going and how to get there. The more populist contemporary bereavement literature belongs within the genre of psychological self-help books, long fashionable in North America and now increasingly so elsewhere in the West.

> Conceiving of solutions to problems – even life itself – as simplifiable into numbered steps, or discrete natural phases, has been a staple of this genre . . . Self-help authors seek to make thoughts and actions make sense. In self-help books this has always meant divvying up events and emotions into categories, arranging them in chronological order, and offering an ideal process for emotional progress.
>
> (Simonds and Rothman 1992: 161)

In this genre, stages and phases that researchers had originally used in order to *describe* complex data are reformulated as *prescriptions*. Instead of being a more-or-less good description of how people experience grief, they become a set of guidelines for how they *should* experience grief. (See the second quote at the start of this chapter, by a family doctor writing for lay people in a popular magazine.)

Certainly some mourners accept stage theory. A rare and therefore valuable participant observation study found that widows' groups in Arizona, with members mainly aged 50–70-years-old, embraced the idea of a grief process with clear stages:

> I suggested that the grief process they were discussing might be too rigid and that perhaps not everyone follows every step in order. 'There's always someone who wants to be an expert,' retorted one woman. 'You can tell you've never been through it,' said another.
>
> (Wambach 1985: 204)

'The grief process' and 'the stages of grief' were for them a fact, not a construct used by researchers, practitioners and mourners to make some sense of the complex and changing emotions of grief. Wambach found, however, that the widows used 'the grief process' in two very different ways. Some used it as a timetable by which they could judge how they were getting on, rather like anxious mothers compare their baby's development with 'the norm' as found in baby books and child care clinics (cf Lopata 1979: 257). The board members who oversaw the groups also operated with a timetable, being concerned if a widow had not moved on after 12– 18 months. Professionally run groups cannot go on for ever: they may be in high demand, with new mourners needing to join, and resources (both money and staff) may be in short supply so that the number of groups cannot expand indefinitely. In such a situation of supply and demand, the notion of grief being time-limited fits the requirements of the organization that groups also be time-limited.[4]

On the other hand, some widows used the grief process as a *guide* to what might change over time, but without designating a fixed timetable. This induced rather more comfort, and less anxiety about 'how they were doing'. In my observation, the grief process and the stages of grief are taught to practitioners very much as a guide rather than as a timetable. They are intended to enable practitioners to identify the normality of particular reactions, but it is hardly surprising if the guide gets transformed – by managers, practitioners or clients – into a timetable. Wambach also found that her widows attributed the discovery of the grief process to Kübler-Ross, unaware that the research in which she developed her five stages was into dying rather than bereavement. When, in my own teaching, I ask nurses or social workers what they have previously learnt on bereavement, the answer is invariably Kübler-Ross's five stages.

Many mourners reject stage theory. It is remarkable how many do so on the grounds that their own grief has not progressed in a simple unilinear path – they seem unaware that all the leading stage theorists agree with them on this!

> I've read all that stages of grief stuff. I've read everything on death and dying. I can relate to what they say but none of it is me. Mothers don't get over their grief. They don't do it in stages. You just cross over and go back. It's like a circle, when you go round it once, you go back round it again. You do your own thing.
> (White, working-class mother, quoted in Cline 1996: 193)

Mourners such as this have either been sold a travesty of stage theory by an intermediary (an article in a woman's magazine, a doctor, or another bereaved person), or they themselves have read an account of stage theory that does highlight the lack of any simple progression, but at the time the reader was so desperate for clear guidelines that they read simple progression into the text when none was there. The map they thus created in their minds was subsequently disconfirmed by their own experience.

I will be interested to observe to what extent clinical lore embraces Stroebe and Schut's (1999) dual process model of grief. In this model, bereavement entails oscillating between executing new practical tasks and going deeply into the pain of loss, two states which cannot easily coincide. It is impossible to bowdlerize this model into neat unilinear stages. The model also indicates that those not showing grief need not be 'in denial' or failing to go through the stages properly; rather the loss may simply have left them with too many practical tasks on hand for the time being, and they will go back to feeling the pain in due course. If this model is embraced, it may well mark the beginning of the end of timetabling. On the other hand, for this very reason, it may perhaps never become as heartily endorsed as the notion of stages and phases.

Normal and pathological grief

Middleton *et al.* (1993: 44) observe that 'In many areas of medicine it is difficult to distinguish normal and abnormal, non-pathological and patholo-gical, or health and disease. The study of bereavement shares this difficulty.' The problems with the concept of 'abnormal' or 'pathological' grief has led to a proliferation of alternative terms whose authors consider them more useful, for example: absent, complicated, distorted, morbid, maladaptive, truncated, atypical, intensified and prolonged, unresolved, neurotic, dys-functional. Since none of these has won the day, and none can be easily defined and operationalized (Rodgers and Cowles 1991), 'abnormal' and 'pathological' remain in frequent use, even though these two terms are equally problematic to define and operationalize (Stroebe *et al.* in press). Klass (1988: 174–7) found that what a number of respected authors consider psychologically pathological is among bereaved parents statistically normal; it may also be psychologically healthy. Hogan and Greenfield (1991: 98–9) point out that the criteria for dysfunctional grief listed by *The Pocket Guide to Nursing Diagnosis* (Kim *et al.* 1987: 22) are virtually identical to those listed for uncomplicated grief by *The Diagnostic and Statistical Manual* of the American Psychiatric Association (1987). Nevertheless, Middleton *et al.* (1993: 49) are sympathetic to the widespread view among researchers and practitioners that 'some criteria must be developed by which there are common understandings of what is meant by normal and pathological grief'.

The question needs to be asked, why? Why do we need to know what grief is normal and what abnormal? Who needs to know this? Is this a requirement of clients, of culture in general, or of medicine in particular? It is significant that Middleton *et al.* are psychiatrists. Psychiatrists and other highly trained practitioners are in short supply, and they cannot see every Tom, Dick and Harriet who is bereaved. There must be criteria for distin-guishing those who need scarce and expensive therapy from those who do not. At a less rarefied level, the same principle operates when it comes to who is to receive counselling. One family doctor writes 'I do some basic counselling myself but I refer more complicated cases to Cruse' (Porter 1996). Dr Porter uses the concept of 'complicated' grief to justify sending some of his patients and not others for more extended counselling. Like-wise there needs to be some notion of resolution, or healthy grieving, if practitioners are to know when a client no longer needs professional help. It may be no coincidence that some person-centred counsellors not only let the client make this decision, but also eschew the concepts of 'normal' and 'abnormal'.

What this means is that the concepts 'normal grief' and 'abnormal grief', whether or not they relate to anything within clients, certainly relate to the needs of organizations providing bereavement services. Enter here, popular culture. We have already seen (in Chapters 2 and 8) that there are popular criteria for how long people should grieve, and how expressive or contained their grief should be. Every culture polices grief and every culture has norms as to what is acceptable mourning behaviour. In practice, clinical lore's notion of abnormal grief is grief that goes on too long or never begins and grief that is either too much or too little expressed. These are precisely the criteria by which popular Anglo/American culture judges grief.

In sum then, for organizational reasons of supply and demand of services, clinical lore needs to differentiate abnormal from normal grief. Even though this is a conceptual minefield, clinical lore draws on both clinical practice, research and popular cultural ideas of abnormality to create its own, ill-defined but intuitively-plausible, notions of what is normal and what abnormal. From the client's point of view, some are relieved to find that the symptoms they feared were signs of madness are actually normal features of bereavement. Others, though, who are clinically depressed, are afraid to ask for help because they think it normal to be very depressed after a bereavement. The negotiation of normality between experts, popular culture and bereaved individuals is an ongoing feature of the social world of bereavement.

Conclusion: heroic grief?

Seale (1995) has documented the increasing prevalence of a heroic script for the dying – one in which they display courage through being aware and expressive, which in turn allows others to display care and concern. This script, he argues (pp.610–11), is 'particularly suited to the conditions of late modernity, where the project of self-awareness is a central pre-occupation.' Clinical lore, I suggest, opens up the possibility of a comparably heroic grief. The contemporary heroic mourner finds the courage to explore and express her painful feelings, reflexively monitors her progress along a path of pilgrimage well-worn by the feet of countless other pilgrims and, fortified by their tales, eventually arrives at the goal of healing and resolution from which she can return safely to everyday life, a changed woman who has grown through the experience. Once returned, like many a true pilgrim, she regales others on the way with her adventures.

It is not just chance that so many people (mis)identify Kübler-Ross as the high priestess of grief's clinical lore, because her portrayal of heroic dying is indeed very similar to heroic grieving. The stables from which they emanate

– palliative care and bereavement care – have much in common (institutionally as well as conceptually). Both scripts challenge the more private, less open scripts of dying and grieving that had hitherto dominated Anglo/American cultures.

But how many mourners actually embrace this script of heroic, open grief? How many find it helpful to order their chaotic lives according to the stages and schedules of clinical lore? Certainly the widows in Wambach's groups did, and doubtless many others find that the inner psychological logic of 'the grief process' functions to staunch the anomie left behind by the loss of Victorian social mourning. But many of those who join mutual-help groups do so because they reject not only the scripts provided by popular culture, but also those provided by clinical lore. Many other mourners, but a decreasing number, are still unaware of the clinical lore of bereavement. Others may be aware of it, but do not describe their own grief in its terms. Very few of the writings of the (better than averagely educated) panel who responded to the Mass Observation directive of the early 1990s that asked about death and bereavement reflect clinical lore.

What, though, of the 'postmodern' stance that disputes the necessity of 'grief work' and that highlights the many and varied ways in which people grieve? Can people mourn without a script? This is the question I return to again and again in this book (and in an earlier book, Walter 1994). No culture before has abandoned all recommendations as to how to mourn. Just as some are now suggesting that postmodernism in general is just a passing fad, so too in bereavement we may find that clinical lore's grand narrative is not so easily deconstructed and discarded. This need not be because clinical lore's narrative is in any absolute or universal sense correct or true, but because it fits the reflexive, highly individualistic period of late capitalism as effectively as social mourning fitted the patriarchal and status-conscious period of early capitalism.

Summary

This chapter has examined various ways in which clinical lore describes, normalizes and regulates the emotions of grief. Central to clinical lore is grief work: the working through of painful emotions, by which process the mourner eventually lets go of attachments to the deceased and resolves the grief in the course of a year or two. This defines normal grief, a heroic process of working through pain and suffering. Various stages in this process have been *described* by researchers and clinicians, but have often been taken as *prescriptions* by student practitioners. Normal grief is difficult to define scientifically, but provides a chart with which bereavement organizations can ration scarce resources and bereaved individuals gain some sense of progress in their painful pilgrimage.

Further reading

Stroebe, M., van den Bout, J. and Schut, H. (1994) Myths and misconceptions about bereavement: the opening of a debate. *Omega*, 29(3): 187–203.

Worden, J.W. (1991) *Grief Gounselling and Grief Therapy*, 2nd edn. London: Routledge/New York: Springer.

Wortman, C. and Silver, R. (1989) The myths of coping with loss. *Journal of Consulting and Clinical Psychology*, 57(3): 349–57.

Questions

1 Look at the three quotes at the start of this chapter. Which do you agree with? What evidence do you have for your answer?
2 Do you have a concept of what is normal and what abnormal grief? On what basis can you justify it? Do you hold this concept as a practitioner, or as one who has yourself been bereaved?
3 Does stage theory fit your own experience of bereavement?

Notes

1 Groups for bereaved people, of course, link the bereaved with one another in a tangible as well as symbolic sense.
2 'Grief work' could be compatible with continuing the bond with the dead: mourners might still have first to work through the pain of the deceased no longer being physically there.
3 By posing the question, I do not mean to suggest that only contentious beliefs need explaining. The sociology of knowledge considers that all beliefs – true, false or unproved – still need their popularity, or lack of popularity, explaining.
4 We may contrast this with rural Greece or with the Middle Ages, where the interest of the church – whose finances and legitimacy depend on the living praying for the dead – requires that grief go on for as long as possible.

10 | Vive la différence?
The politics of gender

It is important to let your grief come out – we are so bad at letting people cry. There are times when it may be inconvenient, grief is no respecter of time or place but keeping everything tight within yourself is not a good idea. Both men and women feel the need to cry, it is not a sign of weakness but a physical manifestation of sorrow.

(From a booklet given by a major funeral chain to all its clients, and compiled by a woman, Lindsay-Hills 1996: 15)

It is a woman's capacity for reproduction that also gives her firsthand access to the realm of death, as she becomes more vulnerable to pain and loss than men.

(Caraveli-Chaves 1980: 146)

This chapter will explore the campaign to discourage the containment of grief and to encourage its expression. In particular, I will examine whether this privileges a characteristically female form of grief, and whether this in turn is related to the increasing voice women are finding in society at large.

In palliative care, the campaign for more aware dying in which the dying person is required to speak of his or her feelings, has been construed by some as a battle against the medical establishment (Frank 1995), by others as a battle within it (Arney and Bergen 1984), but in either case the medical establishment's definition of dying is crucial. This is not the case with bereavement. True, for most of the twentieth century, psychiatrists have been presented as experts on the subject and bereaved people in the UK are more likely to visit their family doctor than any other professional,[1] but those promoting a more expressive way of grief are not battling against a medical status quo. Indeed, the value of speaking of feelings has hitherto been part of psychiatric lore. Rather, those promoting the value of expressing grief see themselves as pitted against popular culture and its restrictions on expressing emotion, restrictions policed by friends, neighbours, family members, employers and employing institutions (including hospitals). These, not doctors, are the usual targets in the horror stories to be found in expressivist tracts on bereavement. The main object of attack is not grief's medicalization, but a general culture of containment and control.

Expressivism in bereavement care is part of a wider cultural movement. Ralph Turner (1976) perceives a shift from defining the self in terms of commitment to institutional roles (Riesman's (1950) inner directedness), to the self as an expression of impulses or feelings. Bernice Martin (1981) writing in the UK, like Robert Bellah and colleagues (1985) in the USA, identifies two kinds of individualism that profoundly shape the contemporary world: a meritocratic/instrumental/utilitarian version, and a romantic/expressive version. The former is strong in the commercial middle classes, engineering, politics and science; the latter among those in the professions, arts and social sciences. In addition to these sober academic discussions, there are of course thousands of publications promoting expressivism and a smaller number (e.g. Anderson and Mullen 1998) decrying it. Political leaders such as American President Bill Clinton and British Prime Minister Tony Blair, concerned to identify the electorate's feelings as much as public opinion, also tap into expressivism. Expressivism in bereavement care, therefore, is part of a wider movement and is directed against a culture of containment.

How the two cultures clash at the grass roots may be seen in the following true story, told to me by a middle-aged colleague who is an unashamed container, rather than expresser, of her feelings. A motor bike crashes outside Mary's house and she witnesses the man die in front of her eyes. Over the next five or six weeks, passers-by leave flowers at the scene of the accident, so every time Mary comes out of the house she sees them, her memory replaying the gruesome death. She is not sleeping at all well, and eventually asks her husband to remove the flowers. This highly expressive mourning ritual turns out to be dysfunctional for Mary. She has too many memories, and needs distractions not perpetual reminders. While some want to remember, she wants to forget. We may note in passing that this kind of spontaneous memorialization following tragic death has grown over the past 15 years in both the USA (Haney *et al.* 1997) and the UK (Walter 1991b). But some people's expressiveness can disturb others, just as can some other people's reserve.

Research is increasingly indicating that a person's path through grief owes more to personality and habitual strategies for coping with stress than with any universal 'grief process' (Stroebe 1992–3). We have already seen in the previous chapter that the evidence for the expressivist mantra that everyone must 'work through' the pain of grief is currently being disputed. According to Wortman and Silver's review of the research (1989), as modified by Stroebe *et al.* (1994), there are three emotional paths that contemporary westerners most commonly take through grief:

1 Moving over time from distress to emotional stability.
2 Never showing distress.
3 Staying distressed indefinitely.

Other researchers, however, would want to add a fourth path:

4 Moving over time from not showing distress, to showing it.

I have observed earlier that no society leaves people free to grieve as they will, and it would seem that there is a tendency for each society, or faction within society, to validate just one of these paths, usually the first or the second. Path 1, letting the grief out and getting over it, is promoted in expressivist clinical lore, in contemporary Egypt and rural Greece, and was also recommended in Victorian society for upper-class ladies. Path 2, containing the grief, is validated in twentieth-century popular culture, along with some traditional groups such as the Navaho, the Hopi and the Balinese. Path 3 is rather rare, but was traditionally expected of the upper-caste Hindu widow, for whom immolation on her husband's funeral pyre may have been preferable to permanent exclusion from social life: without her husband, she was nothing and would for ever remain so. I do not know of any society that legitimates path 4, except in the very short run when it is expected that the next-of-kin keep themselves together until after the funeral.

What we are witnessing in Anglo/American society is an attempt by expressivists to shift the dominant norm from path 2 to path 1. If Wortman and Silver are right, they will find resistance, for just as the previous norm of containing distress did not fit the personality of some, so the norm of expressing grief will not fit the personality of others. The research evidence indicates that bereaved people often find it helpful to express their feelings, but there is no evidence to suggest this should be promoted as the *only* healthy way to grieve. Expressivists vary to what extent they make this latter claim (as in the quote with which this chapter began) and to what extent they simply say that those who want to be more expressive should not feel inhibited.

Sexual politics?

We could look at any number of battles in the campaign to proclaim the expressive way as 'the right way'. We could look at skirmishes between the expressive professions and the rest of society, or between younger and older generations, or we could look at how the popular media are increasingly being captured by expressivism. Or we could look at reactions to the death of Diana, Princes of Wales, as a case study of one particular skirmish in the war between expressivists and containers. For example: 'I felt *scared* when I saw all those flowers. It seemed a kind of floral fascism . . . a country patrolled by the grief police' (Maggie Winkworth, in Jack 1997: 18). Also 'Then the touchy-feely fascists got to work and it began to seem that not to feel unqualified grief was somehow a heresy' (John Bradshaw, in Jack 1997: 24).

Instead, I will look at gender. Might it be that the battle between expressivists and containers is in part a battle between males and females? Might it be that the path through grief that has been validated for most of the twentieth century (stiff upper lip, let go, move on to a new relationship) has been a typically male path and that the expressivists who are challenging this are women who, at last, have the courage to speak of their own experiences? If this is the case, are they arguing simply for their voice to be heard as well as men's, or are they arguing that their path through grief (expressive, maintaining the bond) is the healthy way for all human beings, but men have been brainwashed into thinking that they do not have feelings or should not express them? Is there research evidence that men and women grieve in different ways? Such are the questions addressed in the rest of this chapter.

Two feminist studies

The dust jacket of Cline (1996) proclaims her book to be 'the first major study of the sexual politics of death'. Does she then illuminate the sexual politics of bereavement? Cline's feisty analysis is weakened by a false claim, namely 'that researchers in this area were looking at the general population without any gender breakdown' (p.18). This is certainly true of many research fields (including research on dying), while other fields have been dominated by data on males that has been generalized unthinkingly to females, but neither is the case with research on bereavement (Field *et al.* 1997: 9). In fact, the data were at first overwhelmingly based on female grief (typically, premature widowhood), from which general theories about the entire population of bereaved people were made. Parkes's (1972) work is classic: based largely on data about prematurely widowed women, his influential book is termed *Bereavement: Studies of Grief in Adult Life* (not 'studies of grief in non-elderly widows'). Bereavement is one of the very few research areas in which women's experience *has* been taken seriously, to the extent of being generalized without great thought to men too. (The reason for the data's selectivity may lie in the nineteenth-century construction of bereavement as a woman's problem; also, there are many more widows than widowers.) When Cline claims (p.22) that 'women's response to death and dying has been subsumed under men's relationship to death', she may be right for dying, but certainly not for grieving. There, men's grieving has been subsumed under women's.

Cline interviewed 200 women in order that women's voices could be heard. Though this feminist methodology is entirely appropriate in other research areas, in bereavement the most illuminating research would look at men, or compare male grief with female grief (Stroebe 1998). Researchers are currently wondering 'We know how women grieve, but we know very little about male grief.' Many publications on bereavement refer to 'people' when they mean 'women', and thus falsely generalize. Cline, by contrast, refers throughout to 'women', running the opposite danger of falsely particularizing. For example (p.19) 'Many women did not want to be controlled by what is seen as an appropriate time for grief.' Some men also feel this, but the naive reader could well suppose that it is typically women who are controlled in this way. Maybe they are, but Cline's all-female methodology gives her no basis for saying whether or not grieving women feel more controlled than do grieving men. She likewise shows that many women want to maintain their bonds to the dead and that this contradicts major theories of grief, but she is unable to say whether more women than men feel this way, and therefore whether or not this really is a gender issue. Her book is refreshing in taking the policing of grief seriously, but ultimately obscures rather than illuminates how this policing is gendered.

A more promising starting point is an observation made by two other feminists, Simonds and Rothman (1992: 185), in their historical study of consolation literature for mothers whose babies have died. They observe that virtually all late twentieth-century consolation books take it as axiomatic that the father's grief is as intense as the mother's, but he rarely shows it. It seems to me that expressivists assume this of *all* forms of grief: fathers grieve as much as mothers, widowers as much as widows, brothers as much as sisters, sons as much as daughters, only they do not know how to show it. Workshops on men's grief abound and expressivists are greatly exercised about how to help grieving men be more open about their feelings. Simonds and Rothman prompt us to ask what is the evidence that men grieve as much as women, or that they have the same kind of feelings?

Two questions

Silverman's (1986) *Widow-to-Widow* programme originally (1967) tried to recruit volunteer helpers from widowers as well as from widows, but could only get widows to volunteer. Mutual-help groups for bereaved parents typically have many more mothers than fathers. Laura Palmer found that

> While reading through the hundreds of letters and poems that have been left at the [Vietnam Veterans] memorial, I never encountered one

that was written from a father to his son. Sometimes a man would write 'Love Dad' on the bottom of a note from his wife, but rarely was there anything more. Fathers who were at home when I arrived participated in the interviews with eagerness and candour, but they are apparently less inclined to express themselves in writing.

(Palmer 1988: xv)

Palmer found, however, that brothers and pals did leave written messages at the Vietnam wall. One might expect loss of a sibling to be less markedly gendered than loss of a spouse or child. Yet even here we find many more females than males expressing themselves and joining mutual help groups. In my only copy (Spring 1992) of the newsletter of SIBBS (Support In Bereavement for Brothers and Sisters), all nine of the personal accounts and requests to make contact with similarly bereaved children are by females. In Greek and Ingrian cultures, women perform highly expressive ritual laments (Danforth 1982; Nenola-Kallio 1982). A comparative survey of grief in 78 different cultures found that in about half men and women cried equally, and in about half women cried more than men, but in no culture did men cry more (Rosenblatt et al. 1976: 21–7).

How do we explain such differences? Are there real differences between the sexes when it comes to grief? Or can it all be accounted for by the expressivist position that – despite all observable evidence – bereaved husbands, fathers and brothers are nevertheless, deep inside, grieving just as much as the women, but do not know how to show it (and therefore need to be helped to show it)? To answer this I will look at two key questions: (1) Is there evidence that men in the contemporary West grieve as much as women? (2) Is there evidence that men grieve the same way as women? In what follows, I am of course referring only to tendencies and probabilities; there is enormous variation within as well as between genders.

Do men grieve as much as women?

Stroebe's (1998) review of sex differences concentrates on loss of a spouse. When it comes to health indicators such as depression, Stroebe reminds us that widows being more depressed than widowers may reflect the generally higher levels of depression among women, rather than reflecting the loss of their spouse. When these factors are disentangled, the evidence (in the contemporary West, at least) is clear: although widows are more depressed than widowers, the *increase* in depression on bereavement is greater in widowers than in widows. Though widows express their upset more, widowerhood is more likely to lead to depression and earlier death, especially suicide.

Stroebe suggests that this is not entirely surprising. There is considerable evidence that men tend to benefit from marriage more than do women

– wives are often their main or indeed only confidant, whereas wives more often have others, typically other women, in whom they can confide. Consequently, widowers are more likely than widows to be left stranded. (The one exception is remarriage, where middle aged and older men find a much bigger pool of potential partners than do women.) We may conclude that widowers typically suffer a greater loss than do widows, but do not show their pain, which is manifested more in depression, disease and suicide. This fits the expressivist thesis that men grieve deeply and can be helped by counselling or therapy that helps them confront their emotions.

What about other kinds of loss? Although there is no research as carefully controlled as Stroebe's study comparing widows and widowers, research by Cleiren (1991) indicates that in non-spousal bereavement women are more troubled than men and for longer. This seems to be the case for those who have lost a child, and there is clear evidence that sisters tend to grieve the loss of a sibling harder and longer than do brothers.

With miscarriage, abortion and loss of a young infant, it should not be surprising that mothers tend to grieve more than fathers. One does not have to presuppose maternal instincts or intuitive nurturing capacities to observe that women bear babies and men do not. The baby is, or has been, a part of the woman in a way it is not part of the man, so the woman who loses a baby is far more likely to feel she has lost a part of herself (Simonds and Rothman 1992: 184, 252). If the child dies at a somewhat older age, and/or if the father has been heavily involved it its care after its birth, his loss is likely to match hers.[2] Women write most of the published personal accounts of parental loss, and comprise most of the members of mutual-help groups for bereaved parents. Is this because most (though not all) mothers grieve more intensely and for longer than do most fathers? Is it because they grieve a loss of themselves, whereas the men tend more to grieve the loss of another person?

The second quote at the start of this chapter observes, 'it is a woman's capacity for reproduction that (makes her) more vulnerable to pain and loss than men'. In Greece and Ingria (Danforth 1982; Nenola-Kallio 1982), the words of women's laments frequently connect a woman's lot as mother with a woman's role in articulating grief of all kinds. Perhaps it is not just in infant death that women have a particular vulnerability to loss? There is considerable evidence that girls grow up to develop a greater sense of connection to others, as manifested in Gilligan's (1982) finding that girls' moral sense is more concerned with the effects of actions on others whereas boys are more concerned with abstract concepts of justice. In general, males are better at regulation (creating rules, theologies, theories of bereavement), while females are better at integration (connecting with others, pastoral care, bereavement counselling). Losing the connection, through death, may hit a woman harder, or conversely she may have a wider network of people with whom she connects, providing support for any one loss. But either way, the experience of bereavement will be deeply influenced by the depth and range of attachments, which in turn are influenced by gender.

Chodorow (1989), writing from a feminist psychoanalytic standpoint, has proposed an explanation for women's greater ability to connect with others. Both baby girls and baby boys are (usually) closely bonded with their mothers. For a boy to develop an identity as a male, he must differentiate himself from his mother and demonstrate that he is different and separate from her; hence the ever present threat for the boy of being called a cissy, of being deemed effeminate. He has to *construct* his male identity. The girl can develop a female identity, however, by doing nothing, by remaining close to her mother, by helping around the house, by looking pretty like her mother. The boy finds his male self by separating himself from his mother, and is likely throughout life to see 'selfhood' in separation, autonomy and independence. The girl finds her female self through connection to her mother, and is likely throughout life to see 'selfhood' in connection. Whatever one's evaluation of these processes – as regrettable, or as natural and right – there is little doubt that they occur, at least in modern western society and probably in many other societies too. The processes are of course modified in certain circumstances, for example, if the mother works outside the home, if the father takes care of the little baby or if, because of social change, the young woman expects a career but her mother provides no role model for this.

In Chodorow's view, women are more likely to invest their selves in attachments to others, while males are more likely to find a tension between their sense of self and their attachments. As the poet Byron wrote: 'Man's love is of man's life a thing apart, 'tis woman's whole existence.' I argue that this is likely to have significant consequences for bereavement. If bereavement is, as Bowlby argues, the severing of attachments, then – other things being equal, and often of course they are not – women will find the severance a greater wrench than will men. We may, for example, expect females to feel closer bonds to their siblings. The effect is likely to be particularly noticeable following loss of a parent, especially a mother, from whom the daughter may never have quite detached herself, whereas the son's relationship to the mother (or father) is more likely to be that of two separate people. This is born out by Parkes (1995) who found psychiatric problems to be much less common in adult sons than in adult daughters following the death of the mother. On the rare occasions when they did occur, the sons had remained unmarried and there was clear evidence of an unusually intense and/or dependent ongoing tie to the mother. More positively, it is precisely women's attachments to others that provides social support for them when bereaved: women are more likely than men both to grieve hard and to find support in their grief.

Silverman's (1986) study of American widows (aged under 60) was conducted in the late 1960s, when there was very much the idea that women stayed at home to make apple pie and look after the kids. Whereas their husbands located their identity largely in their work, the wives found theirs in their husbands. John Smith is a worker at Ford, she is Mrs John Smith. Silverman found a number of women who worked outside the home; among these, those who also had good friendship and kinship networks managed exceptionally well. With increasing numbers of women defining themselves in terms of work as well as in terms of marriage and parenthood, so we will see more widows of this kind. At the very least, they will not be at a loss (as were some of Silverman's) to know how to fill up the car with petrol. Advice to get back to work as soon as possible, which I have noted earlier was given in the nineteenth century to men, may well be increasingly given to women and there is strong evidence that some diversion from grief is better than no diversion. What affects gender differences in bereavement here is not biological gender, but where identity, skills and emotions are invested.

This is true even of loss of a child, especially if it has lived a number of years. Riches and Dawson (1997) found that the most isolated bereaved parents were those who before the death had been engulfed by the parental role and after the death continued to anchor their identity in this, by now lost, role. This was usually the mother, but some fathers engrossed in parenting also responded this way. Other parents anchored their identity partly in their work role, and were able to repair their shattered identity by building up this role, a strategy that receives support from the wider culture, but one rejected and/or unavailable to those engulfed by the identity of parent.

We may conclude then, with the exception of spousal bereavement, women tend to grieve harder and longer than do men. Two reasons for this have been discussed: (1) mothers who lose babies in the womb or in infancy typically grieve more than fathers because they see the child as part of themselves, and (2) women are more likely than men to invest in significant relationships, whose sundering may be for them a greater wrench. By the same token, however, they have a wider range of close relationships to sustain them after bereavement, particularly, it seems, after loss of a spouse. If to this is added paid work, providing both an alternative identity and distraction from a house full of painful memories, women may cope with spousal bereavement particularly well.

Do men and women grieve differently?

We may hypothesize from the above discussion about identity that women are more likely than men to continue a bond with the deceased. The man with a more autonomous sense of self may be more able to let go of the dead – to be on his own may not attack his sense of self as it does many women's. This may be another reason, on top of supply and demand and men's lack of support from friends, why widowers are more able to re-marry relatively soon after bereavement (and why their daughters may not be able to cope with this). Again, we are not talking here of biological gender, but of how different people construct their sense of self – increasing numbers of women now see themselves as individuals in their own right. What has not been researched, however, is whether there is indeed any connection between lack of sense of self as an autonomous being and main-taining a bond with the dead. Cross-cultural data would be relevant here. Are cultures that forbid relations with the dead the same cultures that encourage individual autonomy? The two certainly worked together in the Protestant Reformation in Europe, and we may note that at the other end of the world Japan is traditionally a culture with a strong sense of group loyalty, little sense of individual autonomy and clear rituals for relating indefinitely to the dead. Within a modern West that overall encourages personal autonomy, boys are particularly encouraged to develop autonomy, while girls have traditionally been discouraged, though that is now changing.

If western males and females may (and I emphasize, may) differ over maintaining a bond with the dead, or about its meaning, what about how they express grief? There is considerable evidence that males have a more contained way of grieving. In Part I, we encountered men who spoke little but who would visit the grave by themselves, and women wanting to talk about their feelings to other family members. Typical is the following quote from an American widow.

> My son worried me. He never talked about his father. He was away at school (college). He came home and without saying a word he took a leave of absence from school and got a job. I was glad to have him around. He did not cry; he did not talk. He just needed to be there. When he decided to go back to school, we were both ready for him to leave. We never really talked about his feelings, but we didn't need to.
>
> (Silverman 1986: 39)

At first she perceives her son's quiet grief as a worry, but later in the quote seems to accept that this is his way and her acceptance of this in turn enables her to feel supported, rather than alienated, by his presence. As we shall see, not all women accept that men might grieve differently and that this might be okay.

A considerable amount of research indicates that males and females tend to cope with stress in different ways (Verbrugge 1985; Belle 1987; Littlewood 1992). Women tend to prefer social support and emotionally oriented styles of coping, while men prefer to be active and to solve problems. (The main exception concerns anger, an emotion which men are more likely than women to express.)[3] Gray (1993) has popularized this research in his best-selling *Men Are From Mars, Women Are From Venus*, and much of what he writes about the differences between males and females is reflected in bereavement. She wants to talk to him about her feelings or just wants him to be there, but he goes off fishing or to the cemetery to think about things by himself. In the case of parental grief, this can create considerable tension between the partners. At best, men 'often see themselves as having responsibility to contain their own grief in order to look after their wives' (Parkes 1996). Or as one study of couples who had lost a baby concluded, 'Mothers and fathers grieve differently, mothers grieve for their babies, fathers grieve for their wives' (Thomas and Striegel 1995).

We might conclude from this that expressing grief is a more typical female response to bereavement, and containing grief a more typical male response. I emphasize that these differences are typical and not found in every case. In her study of widows, Silverman found that among those who coped most effectively were some who had worked from before their husband's death and who adopted coping styles more like men's. They

> seemed to cope emotionally by holding back and finding ways to avoid their feelings. Sharing feelings . . . was not part of their general style of relationship. With widowhood they confronted overwhelming feelings, feelings that they acknowledged but did not dwell on.
>
> (Silverman 1986: 120)

Why the belief that men and women grieve the same?

I have outlined evidence and reasons – other things being equal – for men grieving differently from women and (except in spousal bereavement) less than women. Expressivists, however, typically paint a different picture. In their view, a popular culture of containment discourages the grief that all mourners feel and need to express. The expressivist programme is a gender-free programme in which men and women grieve equally and need to express this equally. How has this programme come about?

First, the nineteenth century identified grief as a properly feminine condition. Simonds and Rothman argue, I think correctly, that this was part of the feminization of family life, of the emotions and of religion that occurred in North America and Britain at that time and that has continued well into the middle of the twentieth century. Women were believed to be – and in large measure were – more pious, family-oriented, emotional and prone to grief than were men. This led to very different expectations being laid on grieving males and females, men being expected to get back to work and master their grief, women being expected to give way to it during an officially imposed period of mourning. The late twentieth century, however, has seen a colossal march of women out of their homes and into careers, not least into journalism, the mass media and politics – their voice is now heard. Among many other things, women are talking publicly about how they grieve. Whereas for over a century the private (female) world has been kept separate from the public (male) world, now there is much more interchange between the two. So the grief we are hearing about nowadays is the grief of upper-middle class, educated women (Simonds and Rothman 1992: ch.1).[4]

It certainly is true that those who inform the modern world about grief – bereavement counsellors, spokespersons for bereavement organizations, and authors of autobiographical accounts of grief – are very largely women. There is an exception, namely psychiatry and academic research into grief. Here there are as many, if not more, influential males as females, with the most influential academic authors (Freud, Bowlby, Parkes, Worden) all being male. Even those researching continuing bonds are as likely to be male (e.g. Geary, Klass, Walter) as female (e.g. Hogan, Silverman). We must remember, however, that psychiatry and academia are in any case very heavily dominated by males, and compared with that baseline, bereavement experts may include a disproportionate number of females (Rando, Raphael, Stroebe, etc.). Most of the data for these researchers, however, comes from grieving women.

I think all this can explain why the voice of grieving women is now heard loud and clear, whether directly, or mediated through (largely female) counsellors or (largely male) psychiatrists and researchers. Since gender is rarely mentioned, one gets the impression that these female experiences are actually universal human experiences. But why do expressivists want to believe that the difference between men and women is not a real difference in quantity and quality of grief, but in the way culture encourages the male stiff-upper-lip?

Here a second argument from Simonds and Rothman (1992: 183–92) may be informative. Before the industrial revolution and modern medicalized childbirth, mothers giving birth were assisted by female kin and by other local women, but then they became isolated as birth moved into the impersonal hospital, and more recently they have been encouraged to rely more on their husbands as partners in the birth experience. So if a woman today miscarries or her baby dies, she may expect from her husband more than most can give. She wants to know that he shares her feelings and hence, Simonds and Rothman argue, the impassioned belief of some modern women that fathers grieve as much as mothers. The father typically does not feel what she feels, so in her disappointment she turns to a mutual-help group of bereaved mothers who have 'been there' and feels what she feels. The women, still wanting to think their husbands are hurting as deeply as they, resort to the 'men have difficulty showing their emotions' thesis. This is more comforting than to acknowledge that within the marriage they are alone with their grief and must look to other mothers to find real fellow feeling. To acknowledge this means to acknowledge not only the loss of their baby, but the loss of their dream of a marriage in which everything can be faced and shared together.

This argument could be expanded, though not so strongly, to other forms of bereavement. Young and Willmott (1975) and Bott (1971) have described the rise of 'symmetrical' marriages in which each partner's social networks decline on marriage, leaving each partner to share activities with and seek emotional support from the spouse. When bereavement strikes, such people look for support chiefly from their partner. A woman who loses her mother might like to think that her husband felt just as deeply when he lost his mother, only being a man he did not show it. She can then imagine he can sympathize and extend his feelings to match hers – otherwise the gap is too big for sympathy (à la Adam Smith) to be offered.

Whatever the reasons, there seem to be increasing pressures on men to grieve as though they were women. A friend (male, in a symmetrical marriage) wrote after reading an earlier book of mine: 'I was intrigued to see the expressive, talking approach to grieving described as female, in contrast to a traditional male approach of ritual acts. I'm sure a lot of men these days would be relieved to hear that the expressive approach may not necessarily be the only one allowed.' If, a few decades ago, many wives were pressurized by their husbands to snap out of it and shape up, we may now be witnessing a reversal in which husbands are encouraged by their wives to show their feelings more – feelings some may simply not have. The policemen of grief are being replaced by policewomen.

In public settings, however, the old male rules of detaching emotions from the workplace still apply to both sexes, and since more women work they are, in this sense, more subject to policing by males.

Things may be different in cultures where gender roles are more clearly demarcated and where women have their own support networks. In rural Greece, for example,

> The men are held back from demonstrations of sorrow and despair precisely in order to balance the feminine role . . . Situated structurally as the stable elements in a ritual which requires their women to move from normal life to the very margins of existence, the men stand solidly in the light of the day, . . . counterbalancing the liminal and numinous experience of their women, and pulling them back from the dangers of too prolonged a contemplation of disintegration within the tomb.
>
> (du Boulay 1990)

The contemporary western ideal of conjugal togetherness undermines such an acceptance of each other's different paths into and out of grief. But mutual acceptance can and does exist in Western Europe and North America, even if not legitimated in the grief literature. One English mother with several remaining teenage daughters wrote to me about how her otherwise all female household coped with their loss: 'My husband has been the solid rock in the background for all his family. But he has never wanted to talk about it.' Her acceptance of the quiet strength he offers may well be premised on his acceptance of the women's emotionality. She respects his desire not to reveal his feelings, whatever they may, or may not, be.

Implications for practice

Research indicates the following: (1) men and women tend to grieve differently, with women being more expressive of their feelings; (2) widowhood typically affects men more than women, yet men do not express their grief; (3) with other types of loss, however, females tend to take grief harder than do males. What then do we make of the fact that most bereavement care is offered by female staff and taken up by female clients? In 1997–8, for example, 76 per cent of Cruse's 26,000 clients and 86 per cent of its 4500 volunteers were female.

Much (by no means all) bereavement care is offered within an expressivist framework, focusing on the client's feelings. This leads me to suggest four possibilities, each being variations on the theme of needs and wants.[5]

1 Women often need emotion-focused counselling

They grieve more deeply and need to express their feelings more than do men. Others in their household often cannot cope with this, so emotion-focused counselling can be a great help in getting a number of women through grief. A few men are helped also.

2 Women often want emotion-focused counselling

Women tend to express their feelings more, and feel good when others acknowledge and affirm their feelings (Gray 1993), so both they and their female counsellors feel good about counselling that acknowledges and affirms feelings. This may or may not reduce the client's long term grief, but is sufficiently satisfying for both sides to keep the process going, especially for those bereavement workers with minimal training and supervision. Mutual-help groups, with *no* training or supervision, are even more prone to perpetuating this female feel-good factor, whatever the long-term consequences.

3 Men typically neither need nor want emotion-focused counselling

Men, grieving less and being less expressive, keep away from bereavement 'care' that they perceive themselves to neither need nor want, and that simply does not understand how men cope with stress. This is felt especially by members of the emergency services and other occupational groups that deal with death and danger through a macho culture of 'we can take it'. Female members of such groups may share this antipathy to counselling.

4 Women do not need emotion-focused counselling, but men do

A fourth possibility is that neither men nor women want what they need. Recent research by Schut *et al.* (1997) found that teaching widows and widowers to cope in the manner generally adopted by the *opposite* gender was associated with the lowering of distress. Thus widowers were encouraged to focus on emotions and widows to focus on practical problems. Widowers might have preferred to be taught to cook than to explore their feelings, but the latter was what they needed. Widows might have preferred to talk about their feelings, but what they needed was confidence and practical guidance in filling in their tax return or seeking employment. Many men will learn the practical skills anyway, many women will find other women to talk to about their feelings.

This fits Stroebe and Schut's (1999) dual process model, in which all bereaved people need to work on both emotional and practical problems. Women tend to focus on the former and men on the latter, so professional intervention should encourage them to deal with the problems they have been avoiding. Schut *et al.*'s (1997) research is potential dynamite for many bereavement organizations that, it implies, have been offering the wrong things to the wrong people. The system keeps going because women like talking to women about their feelings, and men like to stay away from counselling, but overall the system may be ineffective because it gives clients what they want rather than what they need. Cruse's current plans to supplement the counselling that has dominated its work over the past decade with a greater role for befriending (which may include help with practical tasks) is the kind of reform suggested by Schut *et al.*'s (1997) findings.

Before we jump to conclusions, however, a word of caution about Schut *et al.*'s (1997) study. Their research was based on grieving clients who, although not in need of major psychiatric help, were nevertheless experiencing above average difficulties. Whether all males, and all females, would benefit in the way the study indicates is not yet clear. Their research involved only widows and widowers, and we have seen that this is the one form of bereavement in which men are likely to grieve harder and longer than women; having lost their one and only emotional confidant, they may need extra help to express their feelings. Moreover, things are changing. In a generation's time it may be that every female will know how to fill the car up with petrol so that the widow at a loss with practical tasks will become as extinct as the dodo; and the emotionally illiterate male, while unlikely to become extinct, may nevertheless be becoming a rarer breed.

Summary

This chapter examined the contemporary shift toward legitimating emotional expression, asking whether this represents a new stage in grief's feminization. If the nineteenth century identified grief as the domain of women, to be kept within the privacy of the home, the late twentieth century has seen a re-publicizing of grief, which may be connected with the greater profile of women in public life and especially the communication industries. Expressivists assume that men grieve as much as women, only are more repressed. There is evidence for this in the case of loss of a spouse, but in other kinds of bereavement there is evidence that women grieve harder than do men. One explanation for this may be derived from the work of Gilligan and Chodorow on women's sense of connectedness. Why then do expressivists believe that men and women, despite appearances, grieve equally? I proffer an explanation in terms of the historical shift toward symmetrical families in which spouses seek support from each other rather than from same-sex peers, so grieving women need their male partners to feel like them if they are to offer condolences. Finally, implications for bereavement organizations are sketched, drawing on Schut's recent work, which suggests that what both men and women want may not be what they need.

Further reading

Martin, B. (1981) *A Sociology of Contemporary Cultural Change*. Oxford: Blackwell, chapters 2, 9, 10.

Schut, H., Stroebe, M., van den Bout, J. and de Keijser, J. (1997) Gender differences in the efficacy of grief counselling. *British Journal of Clinical Psychology*, 36: 63–72.

Simonds, W. and Rothman, B.K. (1992) *Centuries of Solace: Expressions of Maternal Grief in Popular Literature*. Philadelphia: Temple University Press, chapter 1 and 183–92.

Stroebe, M. (1998) New directions in bereavement research: exploration of gender differences. *Palliative Medicine*, 12: 5–12.

Questions

1 Men's losses are generally less than women's, because they invested less in the first place. Discuss.
2 Describe a grieving couple you are familiar with. How different is each partner's grief? How might they better appreciate their differences?

3 If you are involved in bereavement counselling, would you describe your approach as focused on emotions, on practical problems, or on neither? Does Schut *et al.*'s research prompt you to reconsider your focus?
4 Bereavement organizations tend to normalize female reactions and pathologize male reactions. Is this true of your own organization? Is it desirable?

Notes

1 Despite Freud's warning (1984: 252) against grief being seen as a pathological condition that requires medical treatment.
2 If the new-born is removed to a special care unit after a difficult and premature birth, the parent who bonds with it may be the father rather than the sick and bed-bound mother. A small but significant proportion of very young deaths are of this kind.
3 Campaigning groups following death by murder or road traffic accidents are more likely to be led by men and suffused by an atmosphere of anger (Rock 1998).
4 In an earlier book (Walter 1994), I argued that the increasingly blurred boundaries between the world of private experience and public health provision help explain the expansion of palliative and bereavement care. I did not then see the importance of women's liberation in eroding this public/private split.
5 Psycho-dynamic counselling, with a clear view of necessary 'grief work', typically privileges a client's needs above his expressed wants. Person-centred counselling, with no pre-conceived notions of grief, will privilege the client's expressed wants.

11 Bereavement care

'It's good to talk.'

(British Telecom advertisements, 1990s)

Bereavement care comes in many forms, apart from the support that people give within naturally existing families, friendships and workplaces. In this chapter I discuss mutual help groups and one-to-one counselling, probably the two most common forms of help specially set up for and/or by bereaved people in modern western societies.

In Walter (1994: ch.4), I presented a typology contrasting traditional, modern, late modern and postmodern death. Each type is based on a specific social context (Table 11.1). These four types are related, but not identical, to the romantic, modern and postmodern approaches to grief we encountered in Chapter 6.

Members of *traditional* societies typically live in small settlements in which both the deceased and the bereaved are known, so the mourner daily meets people who knew the deceased. Especially when undergirded by religion, there are likely to be clear expectations as to how the person should mourn. In many such societies, the ancestors play a clear role, though this has not generally been so in Protestant Europe.

Members of *modern* societies, by contrast, typically live in large settlements, only a fraction of whose members will know that I am bereaved. My experience of grief is therefore essentially private. There may, as in urban Victorian Britain, still be social mourning and religious rituals, but my grief is private, indeed it may be required to be hidden behind closed doors. With the abandoning of social mourning, grief becomes potentially anomic (unregulated), with privacy accompanied by an uncertainty both

Table 11.1 The social context of bereavement

	Traditional	Modern	Late modern	Postmodern
Social context	Community	Public versus private	Professional expertise defines private experience	Private experience becomes public
Authority	Religion	Medicine	Therapist	Self
Bereavement experience	Social mourning	Private grief Anomic grief	The grief process Counselling	MHG (mutual help group)
Required language	Ritual	Stoical reserve	Expressive talk	Expressive/narrative talk
The dead	Group ancestors	Privately experienced Publicly forgotten	Let go	Live on in conversation

how to behave in public and about what private feelings are normal. The main professional help available is pills from the doctor.

In late/postmodern societies, there is an interplay between public provision and private experience. As we saw in the previous chapter, women in particular are writing and speaking about their private experiences of grief, and the training of doctors, clergy, and other professionals now includes sessions on bereavement. The experience of the individual now becomes authoritative in a de-spiritualized, de-ritualized, de-socialized understanding of bereavement. At the same time, scientific medicine no longer ignores grief but categorizes and theorizes it, so that the bereaved individual describes his or her own experience with semi-psychiatric terms such as 'denial', 'the grief process', 'recovery' and 'resolution'. Grief is now regulated through these categories and through the possibility of expert counselling and mutual help groups: the grief process replaces social mourning as the framework within which grief is regulated. Insofar as the self is free to define its own grief, so that there is a diversity of voices undermining any notion of a single, universal grief process, we may refer to *postmodern* grief. Insofar as professional expertise dominates, we may refer to *late modern* grief (Walter 1994).

MUTUAL HELP GROUPS (MHGS)

I follow Silverman (1986: 47) in using the term mutual help group, rather than self-help group. In MHGs, help is given as much as received and the process is mutual in a way that quietly reading a self-help book is not. MHGs come in at least four varieties. First there are those whose relatives died in a common event, whether it be war or a peacetime disaster. Due to the unique circumstances of death, relatives feel they have more in common with each other than with other bereaved people, which may be reflected in the dead being buried together rather than with their families. Examples are war cemeteries and the burial together in Amsterdam of many of the over 300 Dutch holidaymakers who died on 27 March 1977 in the Tenerife air crash. Mutual help groups have formed after many of the disasters of the 1980s and 1990s such as Lockerbie and Hillsborough in which those who were previously strangers feel bonded to each other through their common trauma, forming what Winter (1997) terms a fictive kinship group. Sometimes, as at the Dunblane primary school shooting of 1996, or in ex-servicemen's associations, the members of the fictive kinship group may have known each other before, but became bonded into a unique group through shared trauma.

Second, there are MHGs where those remembered died in totally separate incidents, but the resulting bereavements were all of the same kind, for example, loss of a husband, loss of a child through suicide, loss of a sibling, or loss through murder. Members join because they find that friends and relatives, or even professionals, do not understand this particular kind of loss; members find a bond with other members that makes up for their alienation from friends and relatives. The Compassionate Friends, for bereaved parents, is a classic example of this type; another is the *Widow-to-Widow* programme in North America (though this was not originally set up by a widow).

A third type of MHG, a subset of the second, is where the person has died as a result of the unlegitimated violent action of another, usually murder or a road traffic accident. These MHGs often have a more activist ethos, pushing either to speed up a tardy legal process for the individual member (Klass 1988: 125–38; Rock 1998), or to reform the legal process for the future. (Groups forming after a single terrorist bombing, for example Lockerbie or Oklahoma City, belong to both this and the first type.)

Fourth, there are groups initiated and facilitated by a professional working for a bereavement agency. These are not pure mutual help groups, in that they rely on an outsider to their particular experience of loss, but they may share certain features of mutual help groups. Some groups of type 2 or 3 employ professional advisers (e.g. Klass 1988: 183–92), so the distinction between types 2/3 and 4 can become a bit blurred, but many type 2 or 3 groups are hostile to professionals who 'haven't been there'. So too are some type 1 groups. A leading figure in the Lockerbie support group, who lost her son on the plane, told me how useless counsellors were, and how much better it was to talk to other Lockerbie people. Rock (1998: 143) describes how one speaker told a meeting of Support After Murder and Manslaughter, to murmurs of agreement: 'I was a bereavement counsellor, but until you've lost a child yourself, you know *nothing*!' This self-definition of the group as non- or even anti-professional characterizes not just those MHGs concerned with bereavement:

> Implicit in the self-help thrust is a profound critique of professionalism . . . Traditionally, the professions have been characterized by (1) control of entry into the occupation; (2) colleague rather than client orientation in terms of standards; (3) an occupational code of ethics; and (4) a 'scientific-theoretical' basis for occupational activity . . . The entire ethos of the professional orientation is very different from the self-help orientation which is much more activistic, consumer centred, informal, open, and inexpensive.
>
> (Gartner and Riessman 1977: 12–14)

MHGs rely on experiential rather than professional knowledge or academic research as the way to truth, and the most valued MHG members are those who can use their own experience to handle their own or others' problems (Borkman 1976; Klass 1988: 186).

All four types of mutual help bereavement groups are communities of the bereaved, communities bounded by clear definitions of who is in and who is not. Types 1, 2 and 3 in particular define themselves in terms of a community of experience that is not shared by non-bereaved society, by those suffering other kinds of loss, or by professionals. One bereaved parent who joined The Compassionate Friends (TCF) was not alone in rejecting the 'move on and let go' script she associated with Worden, Bowlby and other authorities:

> I know people think you ought to get over things but I don't see anything to get over. It's part of me, part of what I am. This thing about getting over it I really resent. We went up to a TCF conference . . . and they had a speaker there who was a professional, got no children of her own but she knew everything, and she told you how long it would be before you got over it and she told you the stages of what would happen and that. I really wanted to get up and wring her neck to be honest . . . I found it really, really objectionable.
>
> (Riches and Dawson 1997: 67)

The MHG community is unlike the community of a traditional society. Traditional communities – such as a pre-industrial village – are given by residential proximity and do not need an out-group in order to define themselves. Members know each other in a wide variety of different contexts (work, play, kinship), rather than just one. The mutual help group, by contrast, is a product of modern and late modern society, creating a community of fellow feeling that separates members from the anonymity of mass society, from its professional agents and even from their own uncomprehending families.

What, though, are the social dynamics within MHGs? How do these social dynamics help (or hinder) their members' passage through grief? In what follows, I concentrate on type 2, the type that possibly has the most members at the end of the twentieth century and is typical of a postmodern society in which people turn to strangers with common experiences, rather than to family or neighbours, for their sense of community. Type 2 groups are likely to comprise mainly females. Type 1 groups are more likely to comprise a number of men or – in the case of ex-servicemen's groups – to comprise entirely men.

Communities of feeling[1]

We have seen earlier in this book how many bereaved people, women in particular, find that their feelings are not affirmed by those closest to them. Despite a variety of experiences in the group, MHG members find there people who have been through the same experience and had the same feelings. 'Here at last are people who understand!' This can create a power-ful sense of fusion with the group (Rock 1998), a willingness to disclose painful feelings and to tell a difficult story. In Adam Smith's terms (1759), members do not need imaginatively to stretch their feelings in order to understand, so sympathy is likely to be there in full measure.

> The only people, with a few much valued exceptions, with whom I have felt comfortable revealing my feelings about Simon have been other bereaved parents. With them I experience true empathy and ac-ceptance. No bereaved parent has ever indicated to me that the time for painful feelings should be over . . . Stage models and frameworks of grief like resolution and reintegration have more to do with profes-sionals containing their anxieties than reality.
>
> (Cooper 1991)

Such statements become part of MHG lore.

Different people, however, grieve in different ways, even if they have experienced the same category of loss. A key question, therefore, is whether MHGs can accept a wide range of feeling, or whether the emotions of key members becomes normative. If this happens, as is certainly the case in many type 3 groups (Rock 1998), as many people will be put off as attracted. Parkes *et al.* (1996: 136) comment: 'Some people react to be-reavement by becoming angry; others do not. A mutual help group that has become dominated by angry people will repel those who fear or do not feel anger.' A group norm of appropriate emotion may appeal to one half of a bereaved couple and not the other, so one joins and the other stays away. If the one who stays has his or her response to grief affirmed, and the part-ner's implicitly invalidated, this could worsen communication between them. You are either in, or out, of the community of feeling. Guarding against domination of the group by the emotions and agendas of key members is one reason that some MHGs employ a professional adviser who has wide experience and not suffered the particular category of loss.

A place for the dead

Being asked to describe your feelings, as in some forms of one-to-one coun-selling, can be quite clinical and not at all emotional: you stand outside your emotions looking in, like a detached observer. But being asked to talk about the deceased is a much more emotional business, which may be why family and friends often discourage it. A participant in a widow-to-widow group says 'We can't call our families if we feel like talking about our husbands. They don't want to hear it. They think we'll hurt ourselves by talking about it' (Silverman 1986: 170). A member of The Compassionate Friends says, 'My sister is the worst. She hangs up on me when I mention my dead daughter' (Blank 1998: 36). For many members, the MHG is the one place it is possible to speak of their dead.

Klass (1997) argues that this is central to the chapter of The Compassionate Friends that he has been associated with in the USA. By talking together about their dead children, the children gain a social existence. It can be strangely hard keeping hold of an image of the dead child, especially if friends and relatives are reluctant to talk about him or her. In the weekly or monthly conversation of the group, however, the child gains a socially accredited existence, an objectivity out there beyond the mind of the individual parent. As one parent put it (Hogan *et al.* 1996) 'You all never got to meet (daughter's name), so you get to meet her now. That keeps her alive for this hour – while we are talking about her.' One might go so far as to define the group as the place where the children have a communal existence. Klass argues that after a while, perhaps a few years, the child's social existence in the group eventually enables the parent to internalize the child; at that point the parent may leave the group, so long as the bond with the child can be shared with others at home, at work or in other settings.

Klass's argument is unusual in the psychology of grief in that it recognizes that representations of the dead exist not only internally within the head of a bereaved individual but are also (as any member of an ancestor-venerating tribe could tell us) communally constructed within groups. Indeed, the inner representation may depend on public representation. But, MHGs being late/postmodern temporary groups, the children do not become permanent group ancestors in the way that some adults (rarely children) do in some traditional societies.

Talking about the dead child can be highly emotional. At The Compassionate Friends' meetings studied by Lieberman (1993: 417), the opening ritual of each meeting requires each member in turn to recite the loss of their child, inducing strong emotion in not only the speaker but in the entire group. Lieberman suggests that this may be particularly helpful to men who have not hitherto expressed their feelings and can reunite them with their more expressive wives from whom the death had alienated them. He also notes, however, that this ritual stimulation of emotion can be too much for some, who leave after just a meeting or two, while others may get mired in perpetual grief. Sharing emotions and speaking of the dead are two sides of the same coin: those who cherish this stay, those who cannot stand it leave.

Creating a subculture

MHGs create their own subculture, a culture of feeling in which the dead are the central actors. This subculture is set up in order to provide an alternative to a mainline culture and/or to individual families in which emotion is forbidden and in which the dead may not be mentioned. Mutually disclosing their pain and sharing their children's (or spouses' or siblings') lives enables them to create a story in which they can account for an otherwise senseless loss (Riches and Dawson 1996: 150). This story, or narrative, makes better sense to them than the narratives otherwise available in mainline culture. In the typical MHG story, the dead live on, grief has no end; there is no cure for grief, but grief transforms the person. Words like resolution and recovery are not included in the story. The dominant 'restitution' story told in mainline culture, that bereaved people should quickly restore themselves to normality, is rejected in favour either of a 'chaos' story, which simply acknowledges how awful things are and that there may be no end, or a 'quest' narrative in which the long and painful journey of grief can become a pilgrimage of personal growth and development (cf Frank 1995). Pilgrims are not returned speedily to the status quo ante, but transformed in the course of a long, painful and heroic journey. (This view is of course shared by many professional bereavement workers.)

In some, but not many, MHGs the subculture is one of campaigning for political or legal changes that will either stem the flow of deaths, or bring to book those responsible (Rock 1998). The American group MADD (Mothers Against Drunk Drivers) is an example. In such groups, emotions such as anger are not simply shared, but channelled into political activity. The storyline then becomes: our child will not have died in vain.

People stay with an MHG if the group's storyline fits their personal experience better than do the lines offered outside at work, at home, in society (Shapiro 1994, 1996). But if it does not, as in the example above of someone with little or no anger who felt alienated from the group story, then they leave. The refugee from the world may end up a refugee also from the group:

> When I was ready to talk the rest of the world wasn't. I tried going to Compassionate Friends, but it was a big group that intimidated me. Some had been grieving so long I didn't feel I was in their league. I'd sit there thinking: 'How do they cope? Aren't they good?'
>
> (Cline 1996: 189)

This woman could not identify their journey with her own. Jeanne Blank (1998), having lost her 39-year-old daughter, found the stories told in the local chapter of The Compassionate Friends were not her story. All the other members had lost younger children, and she felt isolated rather than included. So she trawled TCF nation-wide to find other parents of adult children, and wrote a book about their experiences. The tight-knit group that embraces some, leaves others isolated. Some of these may set up alternative groups, catering for a more specific sub-group of the bereaved; as Rock (1998) puts it, if fusion is one side of the MHG coin, fission is the other.

Schooling grief

MHGs thus not only allow members to express their feelings and tell their stories, they also provide a script. As we have seen (Chapter 8), bereavement in modern society can be anomic: people simply have not been told what grief entails, and the rules for mourning may be conflicting or unclear. In the group, the new member learns from other pilgrims what the path of grief is likely to entail. MHGs play an educational role for those suffering anomic grief (Silverman 1986; Videka-Sherman 1990). As Silverman puts it, widowhood is in large measure the learning of a new social role, that of widow, and who better to learn it from than other widows?

MHGs can give mixed messages about the role of expertise. While hostility to experts who have not themselves experienced this kind of bereavement is common, groups also teach aspects of clinical lore. Wambach's group of widows typically told new members 'Have you heard about the grief process?' and 'There's such a thing as a grief process, you know' (1985: 204). The (American) Compassionate Friends annual report for 1986 uses pseudo-medical language, describing itself as (my italics):

> a self-help organization offering friendship and understanding to bereaved parents. The purposes are to promote and aid parents in *the positive resolution* of the grief experience upon the death of their child, and to foster the physical and emotional *health* of bereaved parents and siblings.

As well as opposing some elements of clinical lore, MHG language also reflects and teaches it.[2]

Who joins MHGs?

I have suggested that people join and stay with an MHG if its story and subculture fits their experience better than the stories and expectations elsewhere. But which sort of people are likely to identify with the MHG story, and which not? Here the work of Riches and Dawson (1997) is illuminating. We have already encountered it in my discussion of gender in the previous chapter, where it was suggested that the crucial difference is not biological maleness or femaleness but the roles and identities that a bereaved person embraces. Riches and Dawson write about bereaved parents, but their analysis could equally apply to loss of a spouse or friend, rather less to loss of parent or sibling.

Slightly adapting Riches (1998), we may note that – like anybody – a bereaved person may be more or less socially integrated and more or less conventional (subservient to group norms). These are, of course, Durkheim's twin dimensions of integration and regulation with which this book began (Figure 11.1).

Figure 11.1   Responses to bereavement

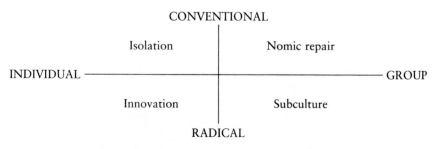

Source: adapted from Riches (1998)

The nomic repairers

These repairers are those whose nomos (view of the world) is repaired through involvement in work and other identities that have little to do with the family that has been shattered by death. These people, chiefly through work, are integrated into society; they conventionally follow the popular culture that encourages mourners (women now as well as men) to distract themselves by throwing themselves into their work. For retired people, social activities or unpaid work may perform this function.

The isolators

These typically do not have paid work outside the home and define themselves in terms of the lost relationship: they are still parents even though the child is dead, still primarily Mrs John Smith even though Mr John Smith is no more. Engulfed in this identity, their connection is so much with the dead that they are cut off from the living.

The subculturalists

Subculturalists are engulfed in the lost identity, but – rejecting conventional advice to immerse themselves in distractions – seek out an alternative society (the MHG) which will affirm, encourage and teach the identity of bereaved parent or widow. 'Bereaved parent', less often 'widow', becomes the master identity, and the group makes it a relatively comfortable identity. Or in campaigning groups, the battle for political change may require decades of voluntary labour, becoming the life project of some members. Some members may find this subculture so enticing that they remain in it indefinitely, not moving on from the group even if they reach Klass's phase of internalizing the dead person – a possibility that professional advisers often warn against.

The innovators

The innovators, accepting that their pre-bereavement identity has been shattered, personally reconstruct their lives in their own way. They are unlikely to join MHGs, or at any rate to stay in them for any length of time.

Riches' framework is insightful because it shows why some people find MHGs helpful, it identifies what some might see as the danger of over-involvement in the group, and it also indicates who are likely candidates for MHG membership. It identifies a common combination: a grieving mother who belongs to an MHG and a bereaved father who is into nomic repair through work. Membership of the MHG may drive such a couple further apart, as her engulfment in the bereaved mother identity is validated by the group as *the* way in which parents mourn, causing her to see her husband's response to grief not as a healthy distraction in work but as a pathological denial of his grief. The problem is that most MHGs do not recognize the validity of those who adopt other coping styles. Another, happier combination (though I make no judgement as to whether it is healthier), is where both partners move from isolation to belonging to a subculture whose group dynamics enable him to construct an emotional self akin to hers.

COUNSELLING

Therapy and counselling have expanded vastly in recent decades as a remedy for all kinds of specific ailments and, in the USA, as an ongoing remedy for life itself. Rose (1989: 227) considers that the rationale of therapy is 'to restore to individuals the capacity to function as autonomous beings in the contractual society of the self. Selves unable to operate the imperative of choice are to be restored through therapy to the status of a choosing individual.' The only duty of the individual is to be free. Giddens (1991), Beck and Beck-Gernsheim (1995) and others write about the burden that accompanies the modern celebration of individual autonomy. It is easier to be told by tradition and other external authorities how to live, how to divide the labour with your spouse, how to grieve; to negotiate these things for yourself requires a much stronger and more autonomous sense of self than that bred in most traditional societies. Therapy (along with progressive schooling, New Age practices and management training techniques) helps the person get in touch with their 'real' self, so that he or she is more able to make choices in the ever-changing world of late modernity.

Rose (1989) does not write (apart from one not very illuminating sentence) about bereavement counselling, but his general argument suggests that counselling finds an affinity with 'letting go' and the 'resolution' of bereavement. The mourner, unable to function as an autonomous being because of attachment to the deceased, discovers through counselling a self apart from the deceased, and thus is empowered to initiate new contractual relationships (in the case of widowhood, a new marriage). But is this what bereavement counselling does? Does it contain a bias toward producing autonomous individuals over and against the communion between the living and the dead that characterized ancestral societies and the European Middle Ages?

Rose is not alone in suggesting that therapy substitutes for many of the functions once played by religion. Indeed, we have already seen that notions such as 'the grief process' and 'grief work', played out within the bereaved's inner psyche have replaced the external mourning behaviours that were required in previous centuries and that often found their ideological base in religion. Even over a period of a few decades, we can observe in the history of Cruse, the UK's leading bereavement agency, a shift from the social, economic and spiritual to the purely psychological (Torrie 1987). Cruse was founded in 1959 by Margaret Torrie, a Citizens Advice Bureau worker, Quaker and pacifist and back then saw widows' problems as primarily social and economic. The first Fact Sheets she produced dealt with income tax, housing, health and diet, pensions, insurance, children's education and training for work. Only later was there a significant shift of emphasis toward psychological counselling.

The early years also saw a determination that caseworkers should have 'a philosophy of life grounded and rooted in spiritual principles'; although preaching of any kind to clients was discouraged, Torrie and her council felt that the newly bereaved sensed in such workers 'a security and certainty they needed when their world had collapsed around them. Kindness was not enough' (Torrie 1987: 20). By the 1990s, though many Cruse volunteers are indeed religious people, it has become an entirely secular organization in which counselling technique and a kind heart *are* seen as sufficient. Knowledge of secular psychology has replaced faith in the eternal goodness of God as the prime requirement. Increasing affluence reduces widows' economic problems, the liberation of women reduces the widow's social isolation and secularization undermines the spiritual basis of care, leaving the client to explore with her counsellor the psychological dimensions of her loss. I do not mean to say that widows have no economic or social problems, or do not believe in an afterlife, but that the processes of affluence, women's liberation and secularization have fostered a counselling approach that focuses on the individual and his or her psychology.

Types of counselling

One important school of thought influencing bereavement counselling is the psychodynamic. Cruse volunteers, for example, have typically undergone a training course, which is highly dependent on this framework, using Bowlby, Parkes and Worden as key texts, although the training is currently diversifying. A study of Cruse counsellors and hospice bereavement workers in the West Midlands in the early 1990s found that they talked to the researcher very much in psychodynamic terms. They talked positively about clients moving through the stages, working through grief and struggling with the pain of loss; and they talked negatively about clients remaining attached to the deceased, not showing their feelings and not being able to let go (Bayliss 1994: 55–6). At the same time, techniques of attentive listening – drawing more on the person-centred approach of Carl Rogers – was also a key part in the training of bereavement volunteers.

Not all bereavement counselling is done by those who come to counselling through a course tailored to bereavement. Some is conducted by generic counsellors who have worked with a range of clients before they began to specialize in bereavement, and who may adhere to any of a number of counselling approaches and schools. Many reject medical models of grief in favour of a companioning model, in which the counsellor accompanies the client on their journey until company is no longer needed.

There is some evidence that, for psychodynamically-trained volunteers, theory does not drive practice. In her questionnaire study, Bayliss found that volunteers saw 'the grief process' as a fact rather than as a more-or-less useful construct (cf Wambach 1985), but when asked to define this process often got stages of grief and Worden's four tasks mixed up. Bayliss wonders whether 'it may be that in their practice the counsellors are actually responding to clients as they find them and not referring to the models at all. Even so, . . . they *see* themselves as using the models, particularly to decide when they can finish their work with clients' (Bayliss 1994: 49). In practice, they may simply be acting as one caring human being faced with another one in distress. Another possibility[3] is that, when being interviewed by an academic researcher whom they may perceive as challenging their expertise, volunteers use the language they learnt in training so they can present themselves as professionally trained, but have no need of such language when counselling a distressed client who is only too pleased to have someone be with them in their suffering. These are only guesses, because virtually no research has been conducted into what actually goes on in counselling sessions.

Virtually all bereavement counsellors aim to provide a safe place in which feelings can be expressed and accepted, and to assure the client these feelings are normal and that he or she is not going mad. They see themselves as reflecting back feelings, but psychodynamically trained volunteers are unlikely to have been introduced to the notion of counselling as a process of interpretation in which the client is helped to edit the story of their loss. A questionnaire study of a bereavement counselling service in London concluded that while counsellors are clear that they provide the core conditions of a safe place in which clients can express feelings, . . . (they are) unsure about addressing issues, which are strongly felt by clients, such as the importance for clients of continuing to think about, or having an 'enduring sense' of their deceased.

(Weinstein 1997: 38)

Anderson and Goolishan (1992) argue that therapy leaves clients a space of 'not knowing' within which they can begin to recreate themselves afresh. Hoffman (1988) suggests that the role of the therapist is that of a friendly editor, helping clients to rewrite their self (see also Cochran and Claspell 1987; Reeler 1993). Such models of therapy/counselling are consistent with the analysis presented in Chapters 3–5 here, and could easily be embraced, it seems to me, by bereavement workers. At present, many psychodynamically trained volunteers to whom I have spoken do seem to be helping their clients rewrite their lives, an observation confirmed by Jennifer Hockey, the anthropologist who trained as a Cruse counsellor:

In describing their experience of grief, bereaved people are subjecting their own intense, inchoate emotion and their extensive personal memories to processes of selection and ordering. What emerges are external verbal forms which the counsellor in turn seeks to edit or clarify. The product is an account, existing outside of themselves, which the bereaved person then submits to further processes of interpretation.

(Hockey 1986: 334)

Few of the volunteer counsellors I have talked to, however, see this as the purpose of counselling. Presumably this is because they have been trained to think in psychodynamic rather than in narrative terms, or at least they have been trained to talk to visiting academics in this way!

Bereavement counselling, like mutual help groups, therefore validates feelings and enables the client to tell the story of the deceased so that it has a reality that exists outside of the client, though the importance of the latter may be less readily perceived by the counsellor than by the MHG. The chief area of difference is in the notion of resolution. Psychodynamically trained counsellors aim to help their clients toward 'resolution', a concept that is anathema to many MHGs. The reasons for this are not only ideological, but also organizational.

First, the demand for counselling seems insatiable, and clients cannot be kept on forever, so there is a good organizational reason why after 10 weeks, or 20 weeks, or a year, or some defined period clients should have 'recovered', 'resolved their grief', begun to 'let go' (Wambach 1985; Broadbent *et al.* 1990). Managers may decide to rein in volunteer counsellors who are too nice to their clients and continue for too long. One manager told me it is entirely up to the client when counselling ends, but admitted she had to resist pressure from the management committee and funders to restrict the number of sessions. By the same token, the lack of any organizational reason for members to leave some MHGs can leave professional advisers in despair about members who have belonged for several years and become perpetual mourners.

Second, those British bereavement agencies that are funded as part of the National Health Service are under increasing pressure to demonstrate their effectiveness. Effectiveness can only be calculated if there is some measurable goal toward which treatment is directed, so the whole enterprise becomes increasingly goal-oriented. Whereas self-help groups tend to see the value of their work as self-evident and not requiring objective evaluation,[4] tax-funded agencies are under the opposite pressure: to construct goals that have more to do with competing with physical medicine for scarce resources than with the realities of bereavement. Linked with this is regular audit of all tax-funded services, including bereavement services. This brings us to the question of research into and evaluation of bereavement care.

Evaluation and research

Here there is a problem. Resolution, as defined in the theoretical literature, is virtually unmeasurable. Whether resolution is defined in Worden's (1983) original terms of 'withdrawing emotional energy from the deceased and reinvesting it in another relationship' or in his later terms of 'finding an appropriate place for the dead in one's emotional life' (1991: 16–17), it is hard to see how either could be unambiguously assessed. Less ambitious is to define the outcome of counselling in terms of return to emotional stability or restored social and economic functioning, although we have already seen that the emotions of grief come in waves and measurement at any one point in time may tell us very little. Less ambitious still is to measure levels of psychological and physical health (such as depression and sleep patterns); this is straightforward as a number of scales measuring these are available off the shelf. The danger here, as in any form of audit, is that we end up valuing what we can measure, rather than measuring what we value. Thus, so long as the client is sleeping well, not consuming antidepressants and not visiting the doctor often, they are 'over' their loss. On the other hand, such things *are* valued in their own right. They are precisely the kinds of suffering that caused clients to seek help in the first place.

S. Rubin (1984, 1991–2) asks whether measures of health and functioning correlate with theoretical notions of resolution such as a successful reorganization of the relationship with the deceased? The jury still seems to be out on this one. There is a further problem (Parkes and Weiss 1983: 29–32). The more it is recognized that it may take several years for this reorganization to take place, the more likely other stressors – both related and unrelated to the original bereavement – are to occur in the meantime. Worst of all, researchers are not at present agreed as to how to define successful resolution, which is in any case likely to be culturally variable – a significant factor in multi-cultural societies.

Nevertheless, a number of researchers, for example Parkes and Weiss (1983: 32), consider that wide-ranging scales can be devised that provide some useful information. Given the drive toward 'evidence-based medicine', they could hardly do otherwise if bereavement intervention programmes are to receive funding. Perhaps the most honest way forward, given this political requirement, would be to abandon any idea of measuring resolution and just stick to health measures: are recipients of the counselling programme less likely to consume anti-depressants, sleeping pills or counselling, and less likely to develop chronic disease? In other words, is counselling cost-effective for the health service? Does it relieve suffering?

Outcome or process?

Despite the methodological problems, research into bereavement interventions has concentrated on the outcomes for those at the receiving end of different interventions. Reviews of outcome research (Parkes 1980; Schut and Stroebe forthcoming) suggest that bereavement counselling can be beneficial when a person is experiencing difficulties, but is not required for all bereaved people. Kalus (1998) has argued that there is a danger of the field becoming inward looking, ignoring the more general literature on psychotherapy. This literature indicates that cognitive and behavioural therapies are most effective, while psychodynamic and person-centred approaches have the least evidence for their efficacy (Roth and Fongay 1996). This appears to be bad news for bereavement counselling that heavily employs these last two approaches, though Kalus reminds us that these approaches are also the least easily evaluated. A lack of positive evidence need not mean they are not effective.

In Chapter 6, I introduced Stroebe *et al.*'s (1992) distinction between modernist and postmodernist approaches to bereavement (their 'modernism' corresponding to the 'late modernism' of this chapter). Stroebe *et al.*'s modernism implies a single grief process, expertise which understands it and positivist research that attempts to correlate particular bereavement programmes with 'resolution' or 'outcome'. Postmodernism, by contrast, implies a multitude of paths through grief with no clear end or resolution and might imply a different kind of research into bereavement intervention. Linda Machin of the University of Keele is researching clients' coping styles in relation to the types of therapy offered to them. The starting point is the client, rather than the expertise of the agency and its personnel. The question then becomes not 'which therapies work?' but 'which clients are likely to find which therapies helpful?' Schut *et al.*'s (1997) research into gender differences asks similar questions.[5]

It is striking, however, that virtually no *observational* research has been conducted into the *process* of bereavement counselling. Palliative care, following the doctrine of total quality management to be found now in health and education as well as industry, acknowledges that process should be audited and monitored as well as outcome. For example, there have been a number of ethnographic (qualitative and observational) studies looking at how nurses interact with dying patients. In palliative care, perhaps it is because the ultimate outcome – death – is not in doubt, that what matters is the process of dying and how care affects that. Bereavement care, however, seems to take the opposite view: never mind how it works, just tell us whether this intervention has a better outcome for clients than that one or is better than no intervention at all. Another reason, perhaps, for resistance to process research is that counsellors and therapists perceive the one-to-one relationship with the client as sacrosanct and likely to be disturbed by the presence of an ethnographer taking notes or subsequently asking the client about how she experienced the session. Video tapes of counselling sessions are, however, made for supervisory purposes, and I do not see any extraordinary ethical problems in these also being used, with the clients' permission, for process research. Very fine-grained conversational analysis of HIV counselling has been conducted by Silverman (1996), research which has been used to inform practice; no comparable research has been conducted into bereavement counselling.

Ethnographic research into bereavement *groups*, though unusual, has been conducted (Wambach 1985; Klass 1988, 1997) and has been particularly valuable, with potentially the same effect as ethnographic work in total institutions (Goffman 1968) and in hospital wards (Glaser and Strauss 1965). When routine practices are put under this kind of microscope, practitioners can gain a fresh view of what is going on and begin to ask the crucial question: do we or do we not approve of what the ethnography has revealed? Ethnographic research has played a significant role in changing the way in which institutionalized patients are treated. Until this kind of research is conducted into bereavement care too, practitioners will continue to perceive what is going on through their own professional spectacles. Bereavement counselling is no different in this respect from any other occupation. I would argue the same for my own occupation, university teaching, where direct observation by an ethnographer of my own teaching would no doubt be uncomfortable, but would probably be the single most effective means of my taking fresh stock of how I teach.

In the meantime, my hypothesis is that what goes on in bereavement counselling is not what the textbooks say goes on. In a number of lectures and workshops I have made assertions about counselling based on textbooks and have been told in no uncertain terms by participants that I have it wrong! This suggests that the relationship is not at all clear between the textbooks, training, what bereavement counsellors perceive themselves to be doing, what an independent observer might conclude they are doing, and what clients think is happening. The relationships between these various elements need to be researched if we are to have any reliable information about the process of bereavement counselling (including how training and professional ideologies relate to practice). Such research would also need to compare agencies and personnel that operate with different models of counselling, and clients (of both sexes) who employ different methods of coping. Such research into process would assist bereavement agencies evaluate their counselling and the training of their personnel.

Summary and conclusion

Bereavement care – consisting chiefly of mutual help groups (MHGs) and bereavement counselling – is now a significant part of Anglo/American bereavement. MHGs are of various kinds, but generally see themselves as communities in which experience and feeling may be shared, with members often having had bad experiences with families and professionals who they feel do not and cannot understand. Klass's research into one MHG (The Compassionate Friends) found that the group provides a social setting in which the dead may have a conversational and ritual presence. Riches's research examines MHGs as subcultures, providing only one of a number of ways of dealing with bereavement.

The chapter then looked at one-to-one bereavement counselling, part of a wider counselling movement aiming to help people become more autonomous individuals. Differences between psychodynamic, person-centred and narrative approaches were briefly discussed, before looking at evaluation and research into counselling. I argued that there is mileage in conducting research into the process of bereavement counselling, comparable to the qualitative research that has recently been conducted in palliative care and in HIV counselling.

This ends Part II, on Policing Grief. Although in popular culture bereavement counsellors are sometimes referred to, disparagingly, as 'the grief police', this chapter has suggested more the opposite, namely that counselling and MHGs often function to provide refuge from a society that many bereaved people feel has policed them too harshly. Compared with other cultures in human history, Anglo/American culture probably polices grief less than most, but Anglo/American individualism causes many of us to value personal freedom exceptionally highly and not to want to have our grief policed at all. I discussed in an earlier chapter the recent roots of this in the first women's liberation movement at the beginning of the twentieth century, a movement that rejected Victorian mourning and instituted twentieth-century private

Figure 11.2   Dimensions of bereavement care

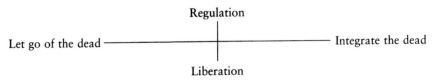

grief, but the historical roots of Anglo/American individualism go back centuries into the mists of time (Macfarlane 1978).

If MHGs and counselling provide a space in which postmodern individualists can explore and share their own unique grief, protected from the policing activities of families and other naturally occurring groups, it is also true that MHGs and counselling produce their own subcultures and their own norms. For those (many) who accept this, the MHG or counselling can be experienced as a blessed relief. Others, however, may become once more a refugee, seeking some place that will let them be themselves.

We may summarize the world of bereavement care in terms of the two dimensions of regulation and integration that run throughout this book. Bereavement care can be, and often is, low on regulation, offering refuge from a society perceived to police bereavement too harshly. But bereavement care can also be quite prescriptive, which may be valued by clients who seek a map of where their grief has got to, but may not be valued by others. This forms the vertical dimension in Figure 11.2. In terms of integration, bereavement care can encourage the client to let go of the dead (as has, at least until recently, often been the case in Cruse); or it can provide a social setting in which the dead can continue to exist (as in The Compassionate Friends). This forms the horizontal dimension of Figure 11.2. The intention behind Figure 11.2 is not to place any one organization of counsellor into a box, but to indicate the terrain within which bereavement care moves. Indeed, any one session of a group or with a counsellor may move quite markedly around this space as clients explore how they wish to relate to the dead and how much freedom they seek for themselves.

Further reading

Klass, D. (1997) The deceased child in the psychic and social worlds of bereaved parents during the resolution of grief. *Death Studies*, 21(2): 147–75. (Reprinted in D. Klass *et al.* (1996) *Continuing Bonds*.)

Lieberman, M. (1993) 'Bereavement self-help groups: a review of conceptual and methodological issues, in M. Stroebe, W. Stroebe and R.O. Hansson (eds) *Handbook of Bereavement: Theory, Research and Intervention*. Cambridge: Cambridge University Press.

Riches, G. and Dawson, P. (1996) Communities of feeling: the culture of bereaved parents. *Mortality*, 1(2): 143–61.

Schut, H. and Stroebe, M. (forthcoming) The efficacy of different types of intervention for bereaved persons, in M. Stroebe, W. Stroebe, R. Hansson and H. Schut (eds) *New Handbook of Bereavement*. Washington, DC: American Psychological Association Press.

Wambach, J.A. (1985) The grief process as a social construct. *Omega*, 16(3): 201–211.

Questions

1 Consider a bereaved person known to you who has moved into (and possibly out of) a mutual help group. Does the analysis of this chapter illuminate their path?
2 Why do you think bereavement counselling and mutual help groups have grown so fast?
3 Measuring resolution of grief is impossible. Discuss.

Notes

1 This term comes from Riches and Dawson (1996).
2 This may be compared to hospices which not only allow people to take control of their own death, but also provide scripts for how this may be done (Walter 1994: Ch.8).
3 Bethan Jones, MA thesis, Dept of Sociology, Goldsmiths College, University of London, 1997.
4 It would in any case be impossible to conduct randomized control trials with MHGs in which members are randomly assigned to different groups (Lieberman 1993). Members must be free to join (and leave) an MHG, and their whole ethos is often hostile to professional or scientific control.
5 Described in Chapter 10.

12 | Conclusion: integration, regulation and postmodernism

This book has addressed two issues in the sociology of contemporary bereavement. The first issue is the social integration of the dead. Bereaved people are positioned between the living and the dead – how do they manage to relate to the dead in a rational secular society that has no place for the dead? The second issue is regulation. All societies control and police the disturbing emotions of grief. How is this done in contemporary western society, and what at present are the fault lines within grief's policing?

Broadly, I identified two positions on the issue of integration. One is that the living must leave the dead behind and move on without them. The other is that the dead are always with us and the bereaved continue to bond with them; indeed the dead must be incorporated in some way if families, other groups and indeed entire societies are to have any sense of their past. Popular culture this century has affirmed both views, though with a definite preference for the former (leaving the dead behind); the latter (continuing the bond) is found primarily in private experience and in public war remembrance. The clinical lore of bereavement experts has reflected popular culture in affirming the former view and pathologizing the latter, though this has begun to change since the late 1980s.

I also identified two positions on the issue of regulation. One is that the emotions of grief should be contained, at least in public, and that distractions are a good way of getting over the pain of grief; this is affirmed by popular culture. The other is that grief must be expressed, talked through, suffered if the mourner is to recover; this is affirmed by clinical lore, and by certain religious and self-help subcultures. Though oscillation theory (Stroebe and Schut 1999) indicates that both may be necessary, when it comes to both popular culture and clinical lore the two tend to be polarized. Table 12.1 schematically depicts the two dimensions of integration and

Table 12.1 Bereavement in Anglo/American culture

| | | Regulation of grief | |
		Contain feelings	*Express feelings*
	Let go of the dead	Protestantism (Ch.1) Popular culture (Ch.2) (including institutional culture, workplaces, hospital wards) 'Male' detachment (Ch.10)	Clinical lore / grief work (Ch.6) Counselling (Ch.11)
			postmodern celebration of variety
Integration of the dead	*Continue bond with the dead*	War remembrance (Ch.2) Private experience (Ch.3) New Age post-secularism	Catholicism (Ch.1) Victorian romanticism (Ch.1) Mutual help groups (Ch.11) 'Female' engulfment (Ch.10)

Table 12.2 Economy and culture

	Nineteenth century	Mid twentieth century	Late twentieth century
Economy	Early industrialism	Triumphant capitalism	Late capitalism
Culture	Romanticism	Modernism: The age of the technical expert	Postmodernism: The authority of the consumer
Bereavement	Continuing bond	Work through grief and let go	Everyone grieves differently

regulation, and how together they produce four combinations. This figure schematically summarizes much of this book.

By the end of the twentieth century, publications on bereavement are increasingly critical of notions of normal and pathological grief, and are emphasizing the variety of ways in which people grieve. Does this reflect a wider postmodern culture that celebrates difference, deconstructs overarching theories and undermines the authority of experts? The 'postmodern' culture of grief accepts that containing feelings works for some people, expressing feelings for others; it refuses to judge whether forgetting or remembering the dead is the more healthy. This is maybe not such a new position: doubtless throughout time there have been tolerant people prepared not to impose their values and coping styles on others. Postmodern culture, however, *requires* tolerance.

Just as Victorian romanticism was a reaction to early industrialism, with home and the emotional inner life being celebrated as antidotes to the horrors of the factory; and just as the modernism of mature capitalism hailed the authority of the rational expert; so postmodernism is rooted in the endless capacity for choice of the educated and affluent consumers who have emerged in late capitalism (Table 12.2). Postmodern consumers of the mass media can choose between hundreds of satellite and cable channels; postmodern patients read up about a range of conventional and complementary cures, and choose their own mix. While public institutions typically generalize, categorize, normalize and pathologize human populations, the private sphere of home and family typically individualizes (Prior 1989); postmodernism sees, to an extent, a higher profile given to personal individual choice. To an extent, popular culture will continue to affirm that 'everyone's different'. Will postmodern mourners, then, flick through a range of bereavement autobiographies, sample some counselling here, a mutual help group there, until they find a support group, a theory, a language that affirms their own experience of grief?

Most will not. Postmodernism is born of affluence and information technology, both of which nurture autonomous individuals who (think they) know their own minds. Most bereaved people are not like that. They are suffering and confused, may not know how they will get through the next day, and are ill-informed about the services on offer. Few, if any, find the bereavement service of their choice by surfing the internet. Like the drowning, they are more likely to cling to the first lifebelt thrown them.

In any case, questions are being asked about the long-term viability of postmodernism: is it possible to have an entire culture based on relativity? Do people and societies not need grand narratives to sustain them through times of change and uncertainty? Will postmodernism – like nineteenth-century romanticism – remain chiefly a movement of artists, writers, architects and other intellectuals opposed to, yet dependent on, the dominant rationality of modernity?

The same may be asked about postmodern theories of bereavement. It is all very well to say that everyone grieves differently, but people need to have some idea of what to expect when they, or others, are grieving. To treat everyone and every moment as unique is not possible, most of the time, and it requires conscious effort (as in person-centred counselling) and/or spiritual discipline (such as Buddhist meditation) if the practitioner is to leave behind years of experience and approach the next client in his or her total uniqueness. Although a few enlightened practitioners may attain this, general attitudes, popular culture and the routine practices of bereavement agencies are unlikely to. In particular, the pressures of accountability will tempt public-funded agencies into generating ever clearer criteria for what constitutes pathological grief and healthy resolution. Postmodern choice is rooted in the power of the affluent consumer, and so I predict that therapists answerable only to private clients, along with a small number of well-funded charities, will be the main sustainers of postmodern grief theories. Acceptance of the wide variability of grief will otherwise, I suspect, remain somewhat marginal, a leisured and romantic voice crying in the wilderness, against both the popular and the expert policing of grief. But I may be wrong. Individualism, in mourning as in so much else, may after centuries a-growing at last have come of age.

LIBRARY, UNIVERSITY OF CHESTER

References

Albery, N., Elliot, G. and Elliot, J. (eds) (1993) *The Natural Death Handbook*. London: Virgin.

Almond, P. (1994) *Heaven and Hell in Enlightenment England*. Cambridge: Cambridge University Press.

Amado, J. (1968) *Dona Flor and Her Two Husbands*. New York: Avon.

Anderson, B. (1991) *Imagined Communities: Reflections on the Origin and Spread of Nationalism*, 2nd edn. London: Verso.

Anderson, H. and Goolishan, H. (1992) The client is the expert: a not knowing approach to therapy, in K. Gergen and S. McNamee (eds) *The Social Construction of the Psychotherapeutic Process*. London: Sage.

Anderson, D. and Mullen, P. (eds) (1998) *Faking It: The Sentimentalisation of Modern Society*. London: Social Affairs Unit.

Ariès, P. (1974) *Western Attitudes toward Death: From the Middle Ages to the Present*. Baltimore: Johns Hopkins University Press.

Ariès, P. (1981) *The Hour of Our Death*. London: Allen Lane.

Armstrong, D. (1987) Silence and truth in death and dying. *Social Science and Medicine*, 24(8): 651–7.

Arney, W.R. and Bergen, B.J. (1984) *Medicine and the Management of Living*. Chicago: University of Chicago Press.

Balk, D. and Hogan, N. (1995) Adolescent sibling bereavement: religion and spirituality, in D. Adams and E. Deveau (eds) *Loss, Threat to Life and Bereavement*. Amityville, NY: Baywood.

Ballard, J. (1996) *One and Two Halves to K2*. London: BBC Books.

Barley, N. (1995) *Dancing on the Grave: Encounters with Death*. London: John Murray.

Barrow, L. (1986) *Independent Spirits: Spiritualism and English Plebeians 1850–1910*. London and New York: Routledge.

Bauman, Z. (1992) *Mortality, Immortality and Other Life Strategies*. Oxford: Polity.

Bayliss, V.J. (1994) How do bereavement counsellors decide that mourning is at an end? an investigation into the models of grief used by those who help the bereaved. Unpublished MA thesis, University of Reading.

Beck, U. and Beck-Gernsheim, E. (1995) *The Normal Chaos of Love*. Oxford: Polity.

Bellah, R., Madsden, R., Sullivan, W., Swindler, A. and Tipton, S. (1985) *Habits of the Heart: Individualism and Commitment in American Life*. Berkeley, CA: University of California Press.

Belle, D. (1987) Gender differences in the social moderators of stress, in R.C. Barnett, L. Biener and G.K. Baruch (eds) *Gender and Stress*. New York: Free Press.

Bendann, E. (1930) *Death Customs: An Analytical Study of Burial Rites*. New York: Alfred Knopf.

Bender, M.P. (1997) Bitter harvest: the implications of continuing war-related stress on reminiscence theory and practice. *Ageing and Society*, 17: 337–48.

Bennett, G. (1987) *Traditions of Belief: Women, Folklore and the Supernatural Today*. London: Penguin.

Bennett, K. (1998) Narratives of Death: a qualitative study of widowhood in women in later life. Fourth International Conference on The Social Context of Death, Dying and Disposal, Glasgow Caledonian University, 3–6 September.

Bentall, R.P. (1990) The illusion of reality: A review and integration of psychological research on hallucinations. *Psychological Bulletin*, 107(1): 82–95.

Bergen, D. (1997) Gender and the 'Unmasterable Past': Memory and mourning in Germany after the Second World War. Conference paper, Mourning, Monuments and the Experience of Loss, Chicago, 16–18 May.

Berger, P. (1969) *The Social Reality of Religion*. London: Faber.

Berger, P., Berger, B. and Kellner, H. (1974) *The Homeless Mind: Modernization and Consciousness*. London: Penguin.

Berger, P. and Kellner, H. (1964) Marriage and the construction of reality. *Diogenes*, 46: 1–25.

Biddle, L. (1998) The inquest system and bereavement by suicide. Unpublished MA thesis, University of Reading.

Biddle, L. and Walter, T. (1998) The emotional English and their Queen of Hearts, *Folklore*, 108: 96–9.

Blank, J.W. (1998) *The Death of an Adult Child: A Book for and about Bereaved Parents*. Amityville, NY: Baywood.

Blauner, R. (1966) Death and social structure. *Psychiatry*, 29: 378–94.

Bloch, M. (1971) *Placing the Dead: Tombs, Ancestral Villages and Kinship Organisation in Madagascar*. London and New York: Seminar Press.

Bloch, M. (1982) Death, women and power, in M. Bloch and J. Parry (eds) *Death and the Regeneration of Life*. Cambridge: Cambridge University Press.

Bloch, M. and Parry, J. (eds) (1982) *Death and the Regeneration of Life*. Cambridge: Cambridge University Press.

Bonanno, G. (forthcoming) The adaptive function of emotional dissociation during bereavement, in M. Stroebe, W. Stroebe, R. Hansson and H. Schut (eds) *New Handbook of Bereavement*. Washington, DC: American Psychological Association Press.

Borkman, T. (1976) Experiential knowledge: a new concept for the analysis of self-help groups. *Social Service Review*, 50(3): 445–56.

Bott, E. (1971) *Family and Social Network*, 2nd edn. London: Tavistock.

Bourke, J. (1996) *Dismembering the Male: Men's Bodies, Britain and the Great War*. London: Reaktion Books.

Bowlby, J. (1961) Processes of mourning. *International Journal of Psychoanalysis*, 42: 317–40.

Bowlby, J. (1969–1980) *Attachment and Loss*, Vols 1–3: *Attachment*, Vol.1, 1969; *Separation: anxiety and anger*, Vol.2, 1973; *Loss: Sadness and Depression*, Vol.3, 1980. New York: Basic Books.

Bowlby, J. (1979) *The Making and Breaking of Affectional Bonds*. London: Tavistock.

Brittain, V. (1933) *Testament of Youth*. London: Gollancz.

Broadbent, M., Horwood, P., Sparks, J. and de Whalley, G. (1990) Bereavement groups. *Bereavement Care*, 9(2): 14–16.

Burns, S.B. (1990) *Sleeping Beauty: Memorial Photography in America*. Altadena, CA: Twelvetrees Press.

Busuttil, A. (1998) Dialogue between pathologists and bereaved after sudden, unexpected death. Fourth International Conference on The Social Context of Death, Dying and Disposal, Glasgow Caledonian University, 3–6 September.

Butler, R. (1963) The life review: an interpretation of reminiscence in the aged. *Psychiatry*, 26: 65–76.

Cadogan, M. and Craig, P. (1976) *You're a brick, Angela!* London: Gollancz.

Cannadine, D. (1981) War and death, grief and mourning in modern Britain, in J. Whaley (ed.) *Mirrors of Mortality: Studies in the Social History of Death*. London: Europa.

Caraveli-Chaves, A. (1980) Bridge between two worlds: the Greek women's lament as communicative event. *American Journal of Folklore*, 93: 129–57.

Carmichael, K. (1991) *Ceremony of Innocence: Tears, Power and Protest*. Basingstoke: Macmillan.

Cathcart, F. and Kerr, J. (1996) Working with death. *Police Review*, 22 March.

Chambers, P. (1997) Why are Most Churchgoers Women? A Welsh perspective. Conference paper, Network for the Study of Implicit Religion, Winterbourne, May.

Childe, V.G. (1945) Directional changes in funerary practice during 50,000 years. *Man*, 45: 13–19.

Chodorow, N. (1989) *Feminism and Psychoanalytic Theory*. New Haven: Yale University Press.

Clayson, A. (1997) *Death Disks: Mortality in the Popular Song*. London: Sanctuary.

Clayton, P.J. (1975) The effect of living alone on bereavement symptoms. *American Journal of Psychiatry*, 132: 133–7.

Cleiren, M. (1991) *Adaptation after Bereavement: A Comparative Study of the Aftermath of Death from Suicide, Traffic Accident and Illness for Next of Kin*. Leiden: Leiden University Press.

Cline, S. (1996) *Lifting the Taboo: Women, Death and Dying*. London: Abacus.

Cochran, L. and Claspell, M. (1987) *The Meaning of Grief: A Dramaturgical Approach to Understanding Emotion*. New York: Greenwood.

Collick, E. (1986) *Through Grief: The Bereavement Journey*. London: Darton, Longman, Todd / CRUSE Bereavement Care.

Cooper, D. (1991) Long-term grief. *British Medical Journal*, 303: 589–90.

Cox, M. and Gilbert, R.A. (eds) (1986) *The Oxford Book of English Ghost Stories*. New York: Oxford University Press.

Cumming, E. and Henry, W.E. (1961) *Growing Old: The Process of Disengagement*. New York: Basic Books.

Curl, J.S. (1980) *A Celebration of Death*. London: Constable.

Danbury, H. (1996) *Bereavement Counselling Effectiveness: A Client Opinion Study*. Aldershot: Avebury.

Danforth, L. (1982) *The Death Rituals of Rural Greece*. Princeton, NJ: Princeton University Press.

Davies, J. (1996) Vile bodies and mass media chantries, in G. Howarth and P. Jupp (eds) *Contemporary Issues in the Sociology of Death, Dying and Disposal*. Basingstoke: Macmillan.

Davies, D. (1997) *Death, Ritual and Belief: The Rhetoric of Funerary Rites*. London: Cassell.

de Hennezel, M. (1997) *Intimate Death*. London: Warner.

Dix, P. (1997) Disaster relief? *Police Review*, 7 November, pp.20–1.

Draper, J. (1967) *The Funeral Elegy and the Rise of English Romanticism*. London: Frank Cass. (First published 1929.)

Dryden, W., Charles-Edwards, D. and Woolfe, R. (1989) The nature and range of counselling practice', in W. Dryden, D. Charles-Edwards, and R. Woolfe (eds) *Handbook of Counselling in Britain*. London: Tavistock/Routledge.

du Boulay, J. (1990) Cosmos and gender in village Greece, in P. Loizos and A. Papataxiarchis (eds) *Growth Points in Greek Kinship and Gender*. Princeton, NJ: Princeton University Press.

Duck, S. (1994) *Meaningful Relationships: Talking, Sense, and Relating*. Newbury Park, CA: Sage.

Duffy, E. (1992) *The Stripping of the Altars: Traditional Religion in England 1400–1580*. New Haven and London: Yale University.

Durkheim, E. (1933) *The Division of Labour in Society*. New York: Free Press. (First published 1893.)

Durkheim, E. (1952) *Suicide: A Study in Sociology*. London: Routledge. (First published 1897.)

Durkheim, E. (1965) *The Elementary Forms of the Religious Life*. New York: Free Press. (First published 1912.)

Dyregrov, A. (1991) *Grief in Children: A Handbook for Adults*. London: Jessica Kingsley.

Eisenbruch, M. (1984) Cross-cultural aspects of bereavement, parts 1 and 2. *Culture, Medicine and Psychiatry*, 8(1): 283–309; 315–47.

Elder, P. (1998) Portrait of family grief, in R. Weston, Y. Anderson and T. Martin (eds) *Loss and Bereavement: Managing Change*. Oxford: Blackwell.

Elias, N. (1978) *The Civilizing Process: Volume 1, The History of Manners*. New York: Urizen Books.

Elias, N. (1982) *The Civilizing Process: Volume 2, State Formation and Civilization*. Oxford: Blackwell.

Elias, N. (1985) *The Loneliness of the Dying*. Oxford: Blackwell.

Erikson, E., Erikson, J. and Kivnick, H. (1986) *Vital Involvement in Old Age*. Norton: New York.

Exley, C. (1998) Last Orders: negotiating pre and after-death identities. Fourth International Conference on The Social Context of Death, Dying and Disposal, Glasgow Caledonian University, 3–6 September.

Farrell, J.J. (1980) *Inventing the American Way of Death, 1830–1920*. Philadelphia, PA: Temple University Press.

Ferraro, K., Mutran, E. and Barresi, C. (1984) Widowerhood, health and friendship in later life. *Journal of Health and Social Behaviour*, 25: 245–59.

Field, D., Hockey, J. and Small, N. (eds) (1997) *Death, Gender and Ethnicity*. London and New York: Routledge.

Finucane, R. (1982) *Appearances of the Dead: Cultural History of Ghosts*. London: Junction Books.

Fischer, C. (1977) Network analysis and urban studies, in C. Fischer *et al.* (eds) *Networks and Places: Social Relations in the Urban Setting*. New York: Free Press.

Floersch, J. and Longhofer, J. (1997) The imagined death: looking to the past for relief from the present. *Omega*, 35(3): 243–60.

Fortes, M. (1965) Reflections on ancestor worship in Africa, in M. Fortes and G. Dieterlen (eds) *African Systems of Thought*. London: Oxford University Press for International African Institute.

Foucault, M. (1973) *Birth of the Clinic*. London: Tavistock.

Foucault, M. (1977) *Discipline and Punish*. London: Allen Lane.

Fraley, C. and Shaver, P. (forthcoming) Theories of grief in contemporary research, in M. Stroebe, W. Stroebe, R. Hansson and H. Schut (eds) *New Handbook of Bereavement*. Washington, DC: American Psychological Association Press.

Francis, D., Kellaher, L. and Lee, C. (1997) Talking to people in cemeteries. *Journal of the Institute of Burial and Cremation Administration*, 65(1): 14–25.

Frank, A.W. (1995) *The Wounded Storyteller: Body, Illness, and Ethics*. Chicago: Chicago University Press.

Frankl, V. (1964) *Man's Search for Meaning: An Introduction to Logotherapy*. London: Hodder.

Freud, S. (1984) Mourning and melancholia, in S. Freud (ed.) *On Metapsychology*. London: Pelican Freud Library Vol.11: 251–67. (First published 1917.)

Gartner, A. and Riessman, F. (1977) *Self-Help in Human Services*. San Francisco: Jossey-Bass.

Geary, P.J. (1994) *Living with the Dead in the Middle Ages*. Ithaca: Cornell University Press.

Geertz, C. (1973) *The Interpretation of Cultures*. New York: Basic Books.

Giddens, A. (1991) *Modernity and Self-Identity*. Oxford: Polity.

Gilligan, C. (1982) *In A Different Voice*. Cambridge, Mass: Harvard University Press.

Gittings, C. (1984) *Death, Burial and the Individual in Early Modern England*. London: Croom Helm.

Gittings, C. (1997) Revenge in a Phone Box: John Soane's mourning for the death of his wife in 1815. Conference paper, 3rd International Conference on the Social Context of Death, Dying and Disposal, Cardiff, April.

Glaser, B. and Strauss, A. (1965) *Awareness of Dying*. Chicago: Aldine.

Glick, I.O., Weiss, R. and Parkes, C.M. (1974) *The First Year of Bereavement*. New York: Columbia University Press.

Goffman, E. (1959) *The Presentation of Self in Everyday Life*. London: Allen Lane.

Goffman, E. (1963) *Stigma: Notes on the Management of Spoiled Identity*. London: Penguin.

Goffman, E. (1968) *Asylums*. London: Penguin.

Goin, M., Burgoyne, R. and Goin, J. (1979) Timeless attachment to a dead relative. *American Journal of Psychiatry*, 136: 988–9.

Goody, J. (1962) *Death, Property and the Ancestors*. Stanford, CA: Stanford University Press.

Goody, J. and Poppi, C. (1994) Flowers and Bones: approaches to the dead in Anglo and Italian cemeteries. *Comparative Studies in Society and History*, 36: 146–75.

Gorer, G. (1965) *Death, Grief, and Mourning in Contemporary Britain*. London: Cresset.

Goss, R.E. and Klass, D. (1997) Tibetan Buddhism and the resolution of grief: the *Bardo-thodol* for the dying and the grieving. *Death Studies*, 21(4): 377–96.

Gray, J. (1993) *Men are from Mars, Women are from Venus*. London: Thorsons.

Gunaratnam, Y. (1997) Culture is not enough: a critique of multi-culturalism in palliative care, in D. Field, J. Hockey and N. Small (eds) *Death, Gender and Ethnicity*. London and New York: Routledge.

Hamilton, M. (1998) *Sociology and the World's Religions*. Basingstoke: Macmillan.

Haney, C.A., Leimer, C. and Lowery, J. (1997) Spontaneous memorialization: violent death and emerging mourning ritual. *Omega*, 35(2): 159–71.

Harrison, R. (1998) Treating trauma. *Police Review*, 22 May, pp.24–5.

Harvey, J. (1996) *Embracing their Memory: Loss and the Social Psychology of Storytelling*. Needham Heights, MA: Allyn and Bacon.

Healy, D. (1993) *Images of Trauma: From Hysteria to Post Traumatic Stress Disorder*. London/Boston: Faber.

Hertz, R. (1960) *Death and the Right Hand*. London: Cohen & West. (First published 1907.)

Hill, S. (1977) *In the Springtime of the Year*. London: Penguin.

Hockey, J. (1986) The human encounter with death: an anthropological approach. Unpublished PhD thesis, University of Durham.

Hockey, J. (1993) The acceptable face of human grieving? The clergy's role in managing emotional expression during funerals, in D. Clark (ed.) *The Sociology of Death*. Oxford: Blackwell.

Hoffman, L. (1988) Like a Friendly Editor: an interview with Lynn Hoffman. *Networker*, Sept/Oct.

Hogan, N. and DeSantis, L. (1992) Adolescent Sibling Bereavement: an ongoing attachment. *Qualitative Health Research*, 2(2): 159–77.

Hogan, N. and DeSantis, L. (1994) Things that help and hinder adolescent sibling bereavement. *Western Journal of Nursing Research*, 16(2): 132–53.

Hogan, N. and DeSantis, L. (1996) Basic constructs of a theory of adolescent sibling bereavement, in D. Klass, P.R. Silverman and S.L. Nickman (eds) *Continuing Bonds: New Understandings of Grief*. Bristol, PA and London: Taylor & Francis.

Hogan, N.S. and Greenfield, D.B. (1991) Adolescent sibling bereavement symptomatology in a large community sample. *Journal of Adolescent Research*, 6(1): 97–112.

Hogan, N.S., Morse, J.M. and Tason, M.C. (1996) Toward an experiential theory of bereavement. *Omega*, 33(1): 43–65.

Holloway, J. (1990) Bereavement literature: a valuable resource for the bereaved and those who counsel them. *Contact: Interdisciplinary Journal of Pastoral Studies*, 3: 17–26.

Howarth, G. (1997) Death on the road: the role of the English coroner's court in the social construction of an accident, in M. Mitchell (ed.) *The Aftermath of Road Accidents*. London & New York: Routledge.

Houlbrooke, R. (1998) *Death, Religion and Family, 1480–1750*. Oxford: Oxford University Press.

Huntington, R. and Metcalf, P. (1979) *Celebrations of Death: The Anthropology of Mortuary Ritual*. Cambridge: Cambridge University Press.

Irish, D., Lundquist, K. and Nelson, V. (1993) *Ethnic Variations in Dying, Death and Grief*. London: Taylor & Francis.

Ironside, V. (1996) *You'll Get Over It: The Rage of Bereavement*. London: Hamish Hamilton.

Jack, I. (1997) Those who felt differently. *Granta*, 60: 9–35.

Jalland, P. (1996) *Death in the Victorian Family*. Oxford: Oxford University Press.

Jalland, P. (in press) Victorian death and its decline, in J. Jupp and C. Gittings (eds) *Death in England: An Illustrated History*. Manchester: Manchester University Press.

Johnson, T.J. (ed.) (1970) *Emily Dickinson: The Complete Poems*. London: Faber.

Jupp, P. (1997) Why was England the first country to popularise cremation? in K. Charmaz, G. Howarth and A. Kellehear (eds) *The Unknown Country: Experiences of Death in Australia, Britain and the USA*. Basingstoke: Macmillan.

Kalish, R.A. and Reynolds, D.K. (1981) *Death and Ethnicity: A Psychocultural Study*. Farmingdale, NY: Baywood.

Kalus, C. (1998) Qualitative approaches to counselling and psychotherapy research. Can they aid our understanding of bereavement care? Conference paper, Bereavement Research Forum, Oxford, 17 June.

Kaminer, H. and Lavie, P. (1993) Sleep and dreams in well-adjusted and less adjusted Holocaust survivors, in M. Stroebe, W. Stroebe and R.O. Hansson (eds) *Handbook of Bereavement: Theory, Research and Intervention*. Cambridge: Cambridge University Press.

Kaplan, L. (1995) *No Voice is Ever Wholly Lost*. New York: Simon and Schuster.

Kearl, M. and Rinaldi, A. (1983) The political uses of the dead as symbols in contemporary civil religions. *Social Forces*, 61(3): 693–708.

Kellehear, A. (1983) Are we a 'death-denying' society? A sociological review. *Social Science and Medicine*, 18(9): 713–23.

Kim, M., McFarland, G. and McLane, A. (1987) *Pocket Guide to Nursing Diagnosis*. St Louis: C.V. Mosby.

Klass, D. (1987–8) John Bowlby's model of grief and the problem of identification. *Omega*, 18(1): 13–32.

Klass, D. (1988) *Parental Grief: Resolution and Solace*. New York: Springer.

Klass, D. (1997) The deceased child in the psychic and social worlds of bereaved parents during the resolution of grief. *Death Studies*, 21(2): 147–75. (Reprinted in Klass *et al.* (1996) *Continuing Bonds*.)

Klass, D. (forthcoming) Developing a cross-cultural model of grief: the state of the field. *Omega*, 39(4).

Klass, D., Silverman, P.R. and Nickman, S.L. (eds) (1996) *Continuing Bonds: New Understandings of Grief*. Bristol, PA and London: Taylor & Francis.

Knight, B. (1997) Death, autopsies and the community. Conference paper, 3rd International Conference on The Social Context of Death, Dying and Disposal, Cardiff, April.

Koppelman, K. (1994) *The Fall of a Sparrow: Of Death and Dreams and Healing*. Amityville, NY: Baywood.

Kübler-Ross, E. (1970) *On Death and Dying*. London: Tavistock.

Kübler-Ross, E. (ed.) (1975) *Death: The Final Stage of Growth*. Englewood Cliffs, NJ: Prentice Hall.

Kuhn, T. (1962) *The Structure of Scientific Revolutions*. Chicago: Chicago University Press.

Lendrum, S. and Syme, G. (1992) *The Gift of Tears*. London and New York: Routledge.

Lewis, C.S. (1961) *A Grief Observed*. London: Faber.

Lieberman, M. (1993) Bereavement self-help groups: a review of conceptual and methodological issues, in M. Stroebe, W. Stroebe and R.O. Hansson (eds) *Handbook of Bereavement: Theory, Research and Intervention*. Canbridge: Cambridge University Press.

Lindemann, E. (1944) Symptomatology and management of acute grief. *American Journal of Psychiatry*, 101: 141–8.

Lindsay-Hills, F. (1996) *Loved and Lost: An Anthology of Words and Poems Dedicated to those who Grieve*. East Grinstead: Funeral Plans Ltd.

Littlewood, J. (1992) *Aspects of Grief*. London: Tavistock/Routledge.

Litwak, E. (1965) Extended kin relations in an industrial democratic society, in E. Shanas and G. Streib (eds) *Social Structure and the Family: Generational Relations*. Englewood Cliffs, NJ: Prentice Hall.

Lofland, L. (1978) *The Craft of Dying: The Modern Face of Death*. Beverley Hills: Sage.

Lofland, L. (1985) The social shaping of emotion: the case of grief. *Symbolic Interaction*, 8: 171–90.

Lopata, H.Z. (1979) *Women as Widows: Support Systems*. New York: Elsevier.

Mandelbaum, D. (1959) Social uses of funeral rites, in H. Feifel (ed.) *The Meaning of Death*. New York: McGraw-Hill.

Marris, P. (1958) *Widows and Their Families*. London: Routledge.

Marris, P. (1974) *Loss and Change*. London and New York: Routledge.

Marshall, V.W. (1986) A sociological perspective on aging and dying, in V.W. Marshall (ed.) *Later Life: The Social Psychology of Aging*. London: Sage.

Martin, B. (1981) *A Sociology of Contemporary Cultural Change*. Oxford: Blackwell.

Marwit, S.J. and Klass, D. (1995) Grief and the role of the inner representation of the deceased. *Omega*, 30: 283–98.

Matturi, J. (1993) Windows in the American garden: Italian-American memorialization and the American cemetery, in R. Meyer (ed.) *Ethnicity and the American Cemetery*. Bowling Green, OH: Bowling Green University Press.

McAdams, D. (1993) *The Stories We Live By: Personal Myths and the Making of the Self*. New York: William Morrow and Co.

McDannell, C. and Lang, B. (1988) *Heaven – a History*. New Haven: Yale University Press.

Macfarlane, A. (1978) *The Origins of English Individualism*. Oxford: Blackwell.

McLaren, J. (1998). A new understanding of grief: a counsellor's perspective. *Mortality*, 3(3): 275–90.

Mearns, D. and Thorne, B. (1988) *Person-Centred Counselling in Action*. London: Sage.

Merridale, C. (forthcoming) *Nights of Stone*. London: Granta/Penguin.

Middleton, D. and Edwards, D. (eds) (1990) *Collective Remembering*. London: Sage.

Middleton, W., Raphael, B., Martinek, N. and Misso, V. (1993) Pathological grief reactions, in M. Stroebe, W. Stroebe and R.O. Hansson (eds) *Handbook of Bereavement: Theory, Research and Intervention*. Cambridge: Cambridge University Press.

Miller, J. (1974) *Aberfan: A Disaster and its Aftermath*. London: Constable.

Mitford, J. (1963) *The American Way of Death*. London: Hutchinson.

Mitscherlich, A. and Mitscherlich, M. (1975) *The Inability to Mourn*. New York: Grove Press. (First published 1967.)

Moore, R. (1975) The spiritualist medium: a study of female professionalism in Victorian America. *American Quarterly*, 27: 200–21.

Morley, J. (1971) *Death, Heaven and the Victorians*. London: Studio Vista.

Moss, M. and Moss, S. (1996) Remarriage of widowed persons: a triadic relationship, in D. Klass, P.R. Silverman and S.L. Nickman (eds) *Continuing Bonds: New Understandings of Grief*. Bristol, PA and London: Taylor & Francis.

Mount, F. (1982) *The Subversive Family: An Alternative History of Love and Marriage*. London: Cape.

Mulkay, M. (1993) Social death in Britain, in D. Clark (ed.) *The Sociology of Death*. Oxford: Blackwell.

Nadeau, J.W. (1998) *Families Making Sense of Death*. London: Sage.

Nash, D. (1996) Look in her face and lose thy dread of dying. *Journal of Religious History*, 19(2): 158–80.

Neimeyer, R. (ed.) (1999) *Meaning Reconstruction and the Experience of Loss*. Washington, DC: American Psychological Association Press.

Nemiah, J.C. (1957) The psychiatrist and rehabilitation. *Archives of Physical Medicine and Rehabilitation*, 38: 143–7.

Nenola-Kallio, A. (1982) *Studies in Ingrian Laments*. Helsinki: Finnish Academy of Science and Letters (University of Turku published PhD thesis).

Newburn, T. (1993) *Disaster and After: Social Work in the Aftermath of Disaster*. London: Jessica Kingsley.

Nickman, S. (1996) Retroactive loss in adopted persons, in D. Klass, P.R. Silverman and S.L. Nickman (eds) *Continuing Bonds: New Understandings of Grief*. Bristol, PA and London: Taylor & Francis.

Okely, J. (1983) *The Traveller Gypsies*. Cambridge: Cambridge University Press.

Opler, M. (1936) An interpretation of ambivalence of two American Indian tribes. *Journal of Social Psychology*, 7: 82–116.

Owen, A. (1989) *The Darkened Room: Women, Power and Spiritualism in Late Nineteenth Century England*. Cambridge: Cambridge University Press.

Palmer, L. (1988) *Shrapnel in the Heart: Letters and Remembrances from the Vietnam Veterans Memorial*. New York: Vintage.

Pardo, I. (1989) Life, death and ambiguity in the social dynamics of inner Naples. *Man*, 24(1): 103–23.

Parkes, C.M. (1972) *Bereavement: Studies of Grief in Adult Life*, 1st edn. London: Tavistock.

Parkes, C.M. (1980) Bereavement counselling: does it work? *British Medical Journal*, 281: 3–6.

Parkes, C.M. (1986) *Bereavement: Studies of Grief in Adult Life*, 2nd edn. London: Penguin.

Parkes, C.M. (1993) Bereavement as a psychosocial transition, in M. Stroebe, W. Stroebe and R.O. Hansson (eds) *Handbook of Bereavement: Theory, Research and Intervention*. Cambridge: Cambridge University Press.

Parkes, C.M. (1995) Psychological problems following the death of a child. *Bereavement Care*, 14(3): 26–8.

Parkes, C.M. (1996) *Bereavement: Studies of Grief in Adult Life*, 3rd edn. London: Routledge.

Parkes, C.M. (1998a) A new paradigm for grief? *Bereavement Care*, 17(2): 28.

Parkes, C.M. (1998b) Traditional models and theories of grief. *Bereavement Care*, 17(2): 21–3.

Parkes, C.M. (1998c) Letter. *Bereavement Care*, 17(3): 47.

Parkes, C.M. (forthcoming) An historical overview of the scientific study of bereavement, in M. Stroebe, W. Stroebe, R. Hansson and H. Schut (eds) *New Handbook of Bereavement*. Washington, DC: American Psychological Association Press.

Parkes, C.M., Laungani, P. and Young, B. (eds) (1997) *Death and Bereavement Across Cultures*. London and New York: Routledge.

Parkes, C.M., Relf, M. and Couldrick, A. (1996) *Counselling in terminal care and bereavement*. Leicester: British Psychological Society.

Parkes, C.M. and Weiss, R. (1983) *Recovery From Bereavement*. New York: Basic Books.

Parry, J.P. (1994) *Death in Benares*. Cambridge: Cambridge University Press.

Pearce, J. (1998) 'Who Asks for a Humanist Funeral?', British Humanist Association, unpublished report.

Pennebaker, J., Rime, B. and Zech, E. (forthcoming) Disclosure or social sharing of emotion: do they help recovery from trauma and bereavement? in M. Stroebe, W. Stroebe, R. Hansson and H. Schut (eds) *New Handbook of Bereavement*. Washington, DC: American Psychological Association Press.

Pennells, M. and Smith, S. (1994) *The Forgotten Mourners: Guidelines for Working with Bereaved Children*. London: Jessica Kingsley.

Peskin, H. (1993) Neither broken hearts nor broken bonds. *American Psychologist*, 48(9): 990–1.

Pike, C. (1983) The 'broken heart' syndrome and the elderly patient. *Nursing Times* 79(9): 50–3.

Pincus, L. (1976) *Death and the Family*. London: Faber.

Porter, M. (1996) On bereavement. *Radio Times*, 12–18 October.

Porter, R. (1989) Death and the doctors in Georgian England, in R. Houlbrooke (ed.) *Death, Ritual and Bereavement*. London and New York: Routledge.

Prince, L. (1996) *Breaking the Silence*. Amityville, NY: Baywood.

Prior, L. (1989) *The Social Organisation of Death*. Basingstoke: Macmillan.

Prigerson, H. and Jacobs, S. (forthcoming) What is normal, what is pathological? A critical appraisal of scientific constructs about bereavement, in M. Stroebe, W. Stroebe, R. Hansson and H. Schut (eds) *New Handbook of Bereavement*. Washington, DC: American Psychological Association Press.

Puckle, B. (1926) *Funeral Customs: Their Origin and Development*. London: Werner Laurie.

Qureshi, H. and Walker, A. (1989) *The Caring Relationship: Elderly People and their Families*. Basingstoke: Macmillan.

Radley, A. (1990) Artefacts, memory, and a sense of the past, in D. Middleton and D. Edwards (eds) *Collective Remembering*. London: Sage.

Reeler, T. (1993) Psychotherapy and story-telling: a Popperian conjecture. *Changes*, 11(3): 205–14.

Rees, D. (1971) The hallucinations of widowhood. *British Medical Journal*, 4: 37–41.

Rees, D. (1997) *Death and Bereavement: The Psychological, Religious and Cultural Interfaces*. London: Whurr.

Ribner, D.S. (1998) A note on the Hassidic observance of the *Yahrzeit* custom and its place in the mourning process. *Mortality*, 3(2): 173–80.

Richardson, R. (1984) Old people's attitudes to death in the twentieth century. *Society for the Social History of Medicine Bulletin*, 34: 48–51.

Riches, G. (1998) Shifting perceptions of the focus in researching bereaved parents. Conference paper, Bereavement Research Forum, Oxford, 16 February.

Riches, G. and Dawson, P. (1996) Communities of feeling: the culture of bereaved parents. *Mortality*, 1(2): 143–61.

Riches, G. and Dawson, P. (1997) Shoring up the walls of heartache: parental responses to the death of a child, in D. Field, J. Hockey, and N. Small (eds) *Death, Gender and Ethnicity*. London and New York: Routledge.

Riches, G. and Dawson, P. (1998a) Lost children, living memories: the role of photographs in processes of grief and adjustment amongst bereaved parents. *Death Studies*, 22(2): 121–40.

Riches, G. and Dawson, P. (1998b) Spoiled memories: problems of grief resolution in families bereaved through murder. *Mortality*, 3(2): 143–59.

Riesman, D. (1950) *The Lonely Crowd*. New Haven: Yale University Press.

Robinson, D. (1995) *Saving Graces: Images of Women in European Cemeteries*. New York: Norton.

Robinson, S.M., Mackenzie-Ross, S., Campbell-Hewson, G., Egelston, C. and Prevost, A. (1998) Psychological effect of witnessed resuscitation on bereaved relatives. *The Lancet*, 352: 614–17.

Rock, P. (1998) *After Homicide: Practical and Political Responses to Bereavement*. Oxford: Clarendon Press.

Rodgers, B. and Cowles, K. (1991) The concept of grief: an analysis of classical and contemporary thought. *Death Studies*, 15: 443–58.

Rose, N. (1989) *Governing the Soul: The Shaping of the Private Self*. London and New York: Routledge.

Rosenblatt, P. (1983) *Tears, Bitter Tears: Nineteenth Century Diarists and Twentieth Century Grief Theorists*. Minneapolis: University of Minnesota Press.

Rosenblatt, P. (1993) Grief: the social context of private feelings, in M. Stroebe, W. Stroebe and R.O. Hansson (eds) *Handbook of Bereavement: Theory, Research and Intervention*. Cambridge: Cambridge University Press.

Rosenblatt, P. (1997) Grief in small scale societies, in C. Parkes, P. Laungani and B. Young (eds) *Death and Bereavement Across Cultures*. London and New York: Routledge.

Rosenblatt, P. and Elde, C. (1990) Shared reminiscence about a deceased parent: implications for grief education and grief counselling. *Family Relations*, 39: 206–10.

Rosenblatt, P., Walsh, P. and Jackson, D. (eds) (1976) *Grief and Mourning in Cross-Cultural Perspective*. Washington, DC: Human Relations Area Files Press.

Roth, A. and Fongay, P. (1996) *What Works for Whom? A Critical Review of Psychotherapy Research*. New York: Guildford Press.

Royal College of Nursing (1995) *Bereavement Care in A&E Departments*. London: Royal College of Nursing.

Rubin, N. (1982) Personal bereavement in a collective environment: mourning in the kibbutz. *Advances in Thanatology*, 5: 9–22.

Rubin, N. (1986) Death customs in a non-religious kibbutz: the use of sacred symbols in a secular society. *Journal for the Scientific Study of Religion*, 25(9): 292–303.

Rubin, S. (1984) Mourning distinct from melancholia: the resolution of bereavement. *British Journal of Medical Psychology*, 57: 339–45.

Rubin, S. (1991–2) Adult child loss and the two-track model of bereavement. *Omega*, 24(3): 183–202.

Ruby, J. (1995) *Secure the Shadow: Death and Photography in America*. Cambridge, MA: MIT Press.

Rutherford, J.F. (1920) *Talking with the Dead?* London.

Ruxton, L. and Miller, J. (1998) The Procurator Fiscal and the bereaved. Fourth International Conference on The Social Context of Death, Dying and Disposal, Glasgow Caledonian University, 3–6 September.

Sarbin, T.R. (1986a) Emotion and act: roles and rhetoric, in R. Harre (ed.) *The Social Construction of Emotion*. Oxford: Blackwell.

Sarbin, T.R. (ed.) (1986b) *Narrative Psychology: The Storied Nature of Human Conduct*. New York: Praeger.

Saunders, C. (1988) Spiritual pain. *Hospital Chaplain*, March.

Scheper-Hughes, N. (1990) Mother love and child death in Northeast Brazil, in J. Stigler, R. Schroeder and G. Herdt (eds) *Cultural Psychology*. Cambridge: Cambridge University Press.

Schor, E. (1994) *Bearing the Dead: The British Culture of Mourning from the Enlightenment to Victoria*. Princeton, NJ: Princeton University Press.

Schut, H. and Stroebe, M. (forthcoming) The efficacy of different types of intervention for bereaved persons, in M. Stroebe, W. Stroebe, R. Hansson and H. Schut (eds) *New Handbook of Bereavement*. Washington, DC: American Pychological Association Press.

Schut, H., Stroebe, M., van den Bout, J. and de Keijser, J. (1997) Gender differences in the efficacy of grief counselling. *British Journal of Clinical Psychology*, 36: 63–72.

Schwartz, B. (1990) The reconstruction of Abraham Lincoln, in D. Middleton and D. Edwards (eds) *Collective Remembering*. London: Sage, pp.81–107.

Seale, C. (1995) Heroic death. *Sociology*, 29(4): 597–613.

Seale, C. (1998) *Constructing Death: The Sociology of Dying and Bereavement.* Cambridge: Cambridge University Press.

Sellars, R.W. and Walter, T. (1993) From Custer to Kent State: heroes, martyrs and the evolution of popular shrines in the USA, in I. Reader and T. Walter (eds), *Pilgrimage in Popular Culture.* Basingstoke: Macmillan.

Shapiro, E. (1994) *Grief as a Family Process: A Developmental Approach to Clinical Practice.* New York: Guilford Press.

Shapiro, E. (1996) Family bereavement and cultural diversity: a social developmental model. *Family Process*, 35(4): 313–32.

Shuchter, S. and Zisook, S. (1993) The course of normal grief, in M. Stroebe, W. Stroebe and R.O. Hansson (eds) *Handbook of Bereavement: Theory, Research and Intervention.* Cambridge: Cambridge University Press.

Silverman, D. (1996) *Discourses of Counselling: HIV counselling as social interaction.* London: Sage.

Silverman, D. and Bloor, M. (1990) Patient-centred medicine, some sociological observations on its constitution, penetration, and cultural assonance, in G. Albrecht (ed.) *Advances in Medical Sociology.* Greenwich, Conn: JAI Press, pp.3–25.

Silverman, P. (1986) *Widow-to-Widow.* New York: Springer.

Silverman, P. and Klass, D. (1996) Introduction: what's the problem? in D. Klass, P.R. Silverman and S.L. Nickman (eds) *Continuing Bonds: New Understandings of Grief.* Bristol, PA and London: Taylor & Francis.

Silverman, P. and Nickman, S. (1996) Children's construction of their dead parents, in D. Klass, P.R. Silverman and S.L. Nickman (eds) *Continuing Bonds: New Understandings of Grief.* Bristol, PA and London: Taylor & Francis.

Simonds, W. and Rothman, B.K. (1992) *Centuries of Solace: Expressions of Maternal Grief in Popular Literature.* Philadelphia: Temple University Press.

Small, K. (1989) *The Forgotten Dead: Why 946 American Servicemen Died off the Coast of Devon in 1944, and the Man who Discovered their True Story.* London: Bloomsbury.

Smith, A. (1759/1976) *The Theory of Moral Sentiments.* Oxford: Clarendon.

Spence, D. (1982) *Narrative Truth and Historical Truth: Meaning and Interpretation in Psychoanalysis.* New York: Norton.

Sque, M. and Payne, S. (1996) Dissonant loss: the experience of donor relatives, *Social Science and Medicine*, 43(9): 1359–70.

Stallworthy, J. (ed.) (1973) *The Penguin Book of Love Poetry.* New York: Penguin.

Stroebe, M. (1992–3) Coping with bereavement: a review of the grief work hypothesis. *Omega*, 26(1): 19–42.

Stroebe, M. (1998) New directions in bereavement research: exploration of gender differences. *Palliative Medicine*, 12: 5–12.

Stroebe, M. and Schut, H. (1999) The dual process model of coping with bereavement: rationale and description. *Death Studies*, 23: 197–224.

Stroebe, M. and Stroebe, W. (1991) Does 'grief work' work? *Journal of Consulting and Clinical Psychology*, 59(3): 479–82.

Stroebe, M., Gergen, M.M., Gergen, K.J. and Stroebe, W. (1992) Broken hearts or broken bonds: love and death in historical perspective. *American Psychologist*, 47: 1205–12. (Reprinted in Klass *et al.* (1996) *Continuing Bonds.*)

Stroebe, M., Gergen, M.M., Gergen, K.J. and Stroebe, W. (1993) Hearts and bonds: resisting classification and closure. *American Psychologist*, 48(9): 991–2.

Stroebe, M., Stroebe, W. and Hansson, R.O. (eds) (1993) *Handbook of Bereavement: Theory, Research and Intervention*. Cambridge: Cambridge University Press.

Stroebe, M., Stroebe, W., Hansson, R. and Schut, H. (eds) (forthcoming) *New Handbook of Bereavement*. Washington, DC: American Psychological Association Press.

Stroebe, M., van den Bout, J. and Schut, H. (1994) Myths and misconceptions about bereavement: the opening of a debate. *Omega*, 29(3): 187–203.

Stroebe, M., van Son, M., Stroebe, W., Kleber, R., Schut, H. and van den Bout, J. (in press) On the Classification and Diagnosis of Pathological Grief, *Clinical Psychology Review*.

Stroebe, W. and Stroebe, M. (1987) *Bereavement and Health*. Cambridge: Cambridge University Press.

Sudnow, D. (1967) *Passing On: The Social Organization of Dying*. Englewood Cliffs, NJ: Prentice Hall.

Taylor, L. (1983) *Mourning Dress: A Costume and Social History*. London: Allen & Unwin.

Thomas, V. and Striegel, P. (1995) Stress and grief of a perinatal loss. *Omega*, 30(4): 299–311.

Thompson, F. (1995) The questions bereaved children ask a doctor, unpublished MSc thesis, Southampton University.

Torrie, M. (1987) *My Years with Cruse*. Richmond, Surrey: Cruse/Bereavement Care.

Troubridge, Lady (1926) *The Book of Etiquette*. Kingswood, Surrey: The World's Work.

Turner, R. (1976) The real self: from institution to impulse. *American Journal of Sociology*, 81(5): 989–1016.

Turner, V. (1977) *The Ritual Process*. Ithaca: Cornell University Press.

Unruh, D. (1983) Death and personal history: strategies of identity preservation. *Social Problems*, 30(3): 340–51.

van Gennep, A. (1960) *The Rites of Passage*. Chicago: University of Chicago Press. (First published 1909.)

Verbrugge, L. (1985) Gender and health. *Journal of Health and Social Behaviour*, 26: 156–82.

Videka-Sherman, L. (1990) Bereavement self-help organizations, in T.J. Powell (ed.) *Working with Self-Help*. Silver Spring, MD: National Association of Social Work Press.

Vincent-Buffault, A. (1991) *The History of Tears: Sensibility and Sentimentality in France*. Basingstoke: Macmillan.

Vitebsky, P. (1993) *Dialogues with the Dead: The Discussion of Mortality Among the Sora of Eastern India*. Cambridge: Cambridge University Press.

Walker, D.P. (1964) *The Decline of Hell: Seventeenth-Century Discussions of Eternal Torment*. London: Routledge and Kegan Paul.

Walter, T. (1990) *Funerals – and How to Improve Them*. London: Hodder.

Walter, T. (1991a) Modern death: taboo or not taboo? *Sociology*, 25(2): 293–310.

Walter, T. (1991b) The mourning after Hillsborough. *Sociological Review*, 39(3): 599–625.

Walter, T. (1993a) Death in the New Age. *Religion*, 23(2): 1–19.

Walter, T. (1993b) Dust not ashes: the American preference for burial. *Landscape*, 32(1): 42–8.

Walter, T. (1993c) War grave pilgrimage, in I. Reader and T. Walter (eds), *Pilgrimage in Popular Culture*. Basingstoke: Macmillan.

Walter, T. (1994) *The Revival of Death*. London and New York: Routledge.

Walter, T. (1995) Natural death and the noble savage. *Omega*, 30(4): 237–48.

Walter, T. (1996a) *The Eclipse of Eternity: A Sociology of the Afterlife*. Basingstoke: Macmillan.

Walter, T. (1996b) A new model of grief: bereavement and biography. *Mortality*, 1(1): 7–25.

Walter, T. (1997a) Emotional reserve and the English way of grief, in K. Charmaz, G. Howarth and A. Kellehear (eds) *The Unknown Country: Experiences of Death in Australia, Britain and the USA*. Basingstoke: Macmillan.

Walter, T. (1997b) The ideology and organization of spiritual care: three approaches. *Palliative Medicine*, 11: 21–30.

Walter, T. (1999a) A death in our street. *Health and Place*, 5(1): 1–6.

Walter, T. (ed.) (1999b) *The Mourning for Diana*. Oxford: Berg.

Walter, T., Pickering, M. and Littlewood, J. (1995) Death in the news: the public invigilation of private emotion. *Sociology*, 29(4): 579–96.

Wambach, J.A. (1985) The grief process as a social construct. *Omega*, 16, 3: 201–211.

Warner, W.L. (1959) *The Living and the Dead: A Study of the Symbolic Life of Americans*. New Haven: Yale University Press.

Warnes, A.M., Howes, D.R. and Took, L. (1985) Residential locations and intergenerational visiting in retirement. *Quarterly Journal of Social Affairs*, 1(3): 231–47.

Weinstein, J. (1997) *My Safe Place: a report on the work of Havering and Brentwood Bereavement Counselling Service*. London: South Bank University.

Weiss, R. (1975) *Marital Separation*. NY: Basic Books.

Wenger, C. (1995) A comparison of urban with rural support networks: Liverpool and North Wales. *Ageing and Society*, 15: 59–81.

White, M. (1988) Saying hullo again: the incorporation of the lost relationship in the resolution of grief. *Dulwich Centre Newsletter* (Adelaide, Australia), Spring: 7–11.

Wikan, U. (1988) Bereavement and loss in two Muslim communities: Egypt and Bali compared. *Social Science and Medicine*, 27(5): 451–60.

Wilkinson, A. (1978) *The Church of England and the First World War*. London: SPCK.

Williams, R. (1981) Mourning rituals: their application in Western culture, in P. Pegg and E. Metze (eds) *Death and Dying: A Quality of Life*. London: Pitman.

Williams, R. (1990) *A Protestant Legacy – attitudes to death and illness among older Aberdonians*. Oxford: Oxford University Press.

Winter, J. (1995) *Sites of Memory, Sites of Mourning: The Great War in European Cultural History*. Cambridge: Cambridge University Press.

Winter, J. (1997) Remembering Total War: forms of kinship and remembrance of the Great War. Paper presented at 3rd International Conference on the Social Context of Death, Dying and Disposal, April, Cardiff.

Wolf, A. (1974) Gods, ghosts and ancestors, in A. Wolf (ed.) *Religion and Ritual in Chinese Society*. Stanford, CA: Stanford University Press.

Wolffe, J. (1999) Royalty and public grief in Britain: an historical perspective 1817–1997, in T. Walter (ed.) *The Mourning for Diana*. Oxford: Berg.

Wood, J. (1977) Expressive death – the current deathwork paradigm, unpublished PhD thesis, University of California at Davis.

Woodburn, J. (1982) Social dimensions of death in four African hunting and gathering societies, in M. Bloch and J. Parry (eds) *Death and the Regeneration of Life*. Cambridge: Cambridge University Press.

Worden, J.W. (1991) *Grief Counselling and Grief Therapy*, 2nd edn. London: Routledge/New York: Springer.

Wortman, C. and Silver, R. (1989) The myths of coping with loss. *Journal of Consulting and Clinical Psychology*, 57(3): 349–57.

Wouters, C. (1977) Informalisation and the civilising process, in P. Gleichmann, J. Goudsblom and H. Korte (eds) *Human Figurations: Essays for Norbert Elias*. Amsterdam.

Wouters, C. (1986) Formalization and informalization. *Theory, Culture and Society*, 3(2): 1–18.

Wouters, C. (1990) Changing regimes of power and emotions at the end of life: the Netherlands 1930–1990. *Netherlands Journal of Sociology*, 26(2): 151–67.

Yamamoto, J., Iyiwsaki, T. and Yoshimura, S. (1969) Mourning in Japan. *American Journal of Psychiatry*, 125: 1660–5.

Young, A. (1995) *The Harmony of Illusions: Inventing Post-traumatic Stress Disorder*. Princeton, NJ: Princeton University Press.

Young, M. and Cullen, L. (1996) *A Good Death: Conversations with East Londoners*. London and New York: Routledge.

Young, M. and Willmott, P. (1975) *The Symmetrical Family*. London: Penguin.

Zisook, S. and Shuchter, S.R. (1986) The first four years of widowhood. *Psychiatric Annals*, 15: 288–94.

Index

abnormal grief, 156, 157–8, 164–5
abortion, 174
accidental death, 94–100
activism, 161
Addenbrooke's Hospital, 99
adolescence, bereavement in, 58–9, 60–1, 87
afterlife beliefs, 57–60
AIDS, 53
Albery, N., 131
ancestors
  in academia, 53
  in Japan, 62, 65, 111
  in modern western societies, 14–15, 61–2, 75
  in mutual help groups, 190–1
  prerequisites for becoming one, 32, 69
  and social death, 50
  street, 74
  threatened by modernity, 110
  in traditional societies, 24–6
angels, 47–8
anger, 160, 190
anomie, 84, 121, 124, 125, 131, 142–3, 150
anticipatory grief, 50
Apache, 26, 41
Ariès, P., 35, 111

atheists' deaths, 85
attachment, 103–7, 175
audit, see evaluation
autopsies, 99

Bailey, E., 61–2
banishing the dead, 22, 26–8, 32–4
Barnardo's, 78–9
Bayliss, J., 197
Beck, U., 125, 195
Bender, M., 40–1
Bennett, K., 84
bereavement
  care, 98–9, 185–204
  counselling, see counselling
  definition, xii
  literature, 145
Bergen, D., 45
Berger, P., 21, 71–2
Biddle, L., 95
Binyon, L., 39
blame, 94–7
Blank, J., 93, 129–30
Blauner, R., 31
Bloch, M., 21
Bonanno, G., 161
Bourke, J., 132
Bowlby, J., 65, 103–6
breaking bad news, 98–9

Brittain, Vera, 43
burial, 48–9
  crisis (nineteenth century), 34
  double, 24–5, 28–9, 38
Burns, S., 63
Byrd, William, 127

Cannadine, D., 44, 142
Catholicism, 128
cemetery, 128
  sculpture, 132
  see also burial; graves
Challenger space shuttle, 31
Chambers, P., 59
Charlotte, Princess, 75
children
  bereavement in, 1–15, 52–3
  protection from parents' grief, 124,
    144, 145
  see also adolescence, bereavement in;
    parent losing a child
Chodorow, N., 175
churchyard, 61–2, 128
Cleiren, M., 174
Cline, S., 123, 163, 171–2
clinical lore, 106–8, 154–6
  elements of, 156–7
closure, 123
Collick, E., 148–9
communities of feeling, 189–90
community size, 30, 73
Compassionate Friends, The, 79, 190–3
complicated grief, see abnormal grief
Cooper, D., 190
coroners, see inquests
corpse, 135
  see also burial
counselling, 10–14, 124, 125, 129,
    195–202
  effectiveness, 199–200
  evaluation, 199–202
  fit of culture and personality, 152
  gender of client, 181–2
  person-centred, 157, 197
  psychodynamic, 197
  and religion, 196
  telling the story of the deceased,
    79–82, 198

terminology used in book, xiv–xv
training, 201–2
translation into language of
  emotions, 158–60
see also Cruse Bereavement Care
courts, 97
  see also inquests
Cowper, W., 127
cremation, 48–9
Cruse Bereavement Care, 155, 159,
    196–8
  gender composition, 181
  history, 196
crying, 134, 143–4
  gender differences, 173

Danforth, L., 24–5
Davies, D., 120
deathbed accounts, 84–102
  early modern, 85
  hospice, 86
  wartime, 88–94
denial, 44, 122, 142
depression, 173
detachment, see letting go
de-traditionalization, 125, 195
dialogues with the dead, 24–6
Diana, Princess of Wales
  beatification, 54
  criticisms of grief for, 81, 97, 147,
    171
  grief for, 21, 31–2, 75, 129, 136,
    150–1
difference, see postmodernism
disasters, 31, 75, 94, 97–8, 123,
    147
disengagement, 38
distractions, 27, 161
doctor, see general practitioner
Doyle, Sir Arthur Conan, 44
Draper, J., 128
du Boulay, J., 180
dual process model, 22, 65, 163–4,
    182
  see also oscillation
Dunblane, 99–100
Durkheim, Emile, xiii, 120, 121, 124,
    125, 129

dying from grief, 58, 173
  thoughts of, *see* suicide
Dyregrov, A., 158

Elder, Kate, 59, 66, 95–6
Elias, N., 126, 153
Eliot, George, 36, 139
emotions, 53, 120–1, 156, 190–1
  celebration of, 112, 132, 148–51
  importance of in modern world,
    xiii–xiv
  inspection of, *see* policing grief,
    regulation
  suppression of, 122–3, 132–4
emotional reserve, 138–40, 143–6
empathy, 129
England, 138–53
Enlightenment, the, 128–9
ethnicity, xi–xii, 49
ethnography, 60, 201
ethnomethodology, 70
ethological theory of loss, 65
euthanasia, 50
evaluation, 199–202
evangelicals, 132
'everywhen', 58
execution, 97
Exley, C., 86–7
expressive grief, *see* expressivism
expressivism, 121, 134, 148–61,
  168–70
  and gender, 178–81

falling in love backwards, 66
family
  fragmentation, 73–4
  relationships, 145, 177, 179–80
  symmetrical, 180
fatalism, 132–4
fear of the dead, 26–8
feminist methodology, 171–2
feminization of grief, 178
fictive kinship group, 43–4, 187
  see also imagined community
finishing business, *see* unfinished
  business
Finland, low cremation rate in, 48–9
First World War, *see* World War One

flowers, 136, 169
forgetting the dead, 40–2, 51–4
  see also banishing the dead
formality, 139–40
Fortes, M., 25–6
Foucault, M., 126
Francis, D., 60–1
Frank, A., 192
Freud, S., 103–5
funerals
  Catholic, 83
  life-centred, 78, 80
  mourners' performances, 144–5,
    148–50
  Protestant, 33–4
  see also burial

gaze, 126, 135
Geary, P., 32–4
general practitioner, 10–11
gender, 171–84
  of grief experts, 179
  see also crying; feminist methodology;
    men; patriarchy; women
Germany, 41
ghosts, 27, 47–8
Giddens, A., 125, 195
gifts to the dead, 27
Gilligan, C., 174
Gittings, C., 33–4, 142–3
Goffman, E., 63, 96
Gorer, G., 139–44
graves
  behaviour at, 60–1
  design, 48
  inscriptions, 51
  tending, 48
graveyard, *see* burial; cemetery;
    churchyard; graves
Gray, J., 112, 177, 181
Greece, 24–5, 174, 180
grief
  complicated, *see* abnormal grief
  counselling, *see* counselling
  definition of, xii
  democratization of, 125, 130–1,
    140–1
  expressive, *see* expressivism

and mental illness, 126
pathological, *see* abnormal grief
as pilgrimage, 165, 192–3
process, 34, 75, 107, 124–5, 197
styles of, 138–53
time-limited, 146–7, 162–3
universality of, 75
work, 103, 160–1
guilt, 96, 121
gypsies, 30

hallucination, 57
Hamilton, M., 26
Hargreaves, Alison, 133
Harvey, J., 72
hell, 47
heroism, 88–94, 165–6, 192
Hertz, R., 24–5, 28–9, 48
Hill, Susan, 121
Hillsborough, 94–5, 147
history, 20, 82
Hockey, J., 159, 198
Hogan, N., 58, 87
Holocaust, 41, 44
homosexual partnerships, 73–4
hope, 57–60
Hopi (Arizona), 26
hospice death, 86
Houlbrooke, R., 85, 127
Howarth, G., 95
hunter-gatherers, 30

idealization, 76–7, 79–80
identity
  family, 72
  gender, 175
  personal, 71–2, 73, 176–7, 193–5
  spoiled, 96–7, 176
  street, 74
  work, 176
imagined community, 43–4, 107
'in memoriam' notices, 51–2, 143–4
inability to mourn, 44–6
individualism, 110–11, 113, 149, 177, 195, 202, 208
inquests, 64, 95, 99–100
integration, xiii, 19–22, 193–4, 203, 205–6

internalization, 66, 105, 191
IRA (Irish Republican Army), 46
Ireland, 139–40, 145–6, 150
Ironside, V., 122, 150
isolation, *see* social isolation

Jalland, P., 132, 134, 156
Japan, 44, 65, 111, 177
  family altar, 62
'Joe Hill', 67
Judaism, 29

Kennedy, John F., 31
Kieslowski, K., 72
Klass, D., 55
  continuing bonds, 105, 106, 109–10
  research with The Compassionate
    Friends, 79, 191
Kollwitz, Käthe, 56, 93–4
Koppelman, K., 71
Kübler-Ross, E., 86, 163, 165–6
Kuhn, T., 108

laments, 174
le Poidevin, S., 158
leisure, 35–6, 208
Lendrum, S., 159
letting go, x, 66, 104–12
Lewis, C.S., 105
Lieberman, M., 191
life review, 101
liminality, 28, 107–8
linking objects, 61–4, 122
Littlewood, J., 66, 84, 147
Lockerbie, 97
Lofland, L., 35–6
longevity, 74
loss of parent, 62, 146–7
  gender of mourner, 175, 180
  see also children

Machin, L., 200–1
McLaren, J., 157
Madagascar, 21
marriage, *see* family
Marris, P., 141
Marshall, V., 101
Martin, B., 169

Marwit, S., 66–7
medicalization, 85–6, 193
mediums, *see* spiritualism
melancholy, cult of, 127–8
memory books, 78–9
men, 61, 171–84
  emotional containment, 177–8
  see also gender; widowers
methodological agnosticism, 68
methods, *see* ethnography; feminist
    methodology; methodological
    agnosticism
Middle Ages, 32
  deathbed accounts, 85
Middleton, D., 164
miscarriage, 174, 179
missing in action, 93
Mitscherlich, A. & M., 41, 44
mobility, geographical, 74
models of grief, 103
modernism, 110–13, 185–7
Moss, M. & S., 76
mourning
  definition, xii
  dress, 131, 135–6, 145
murder, 96–7
music, 52, 127
Muslims, 140
mutual help groups, 79, 98, 124, 130,
    155, 187–95
  campaigning groups, 160, 188, 192
  facilitated groups, 162, 188, 190
  gender composition, 174, 189
  membership, 193–5
  opposed to professionals, 188–90
  subculture, 191–2
  telling the story of the deceased,
    190–1
  types of, 187–9

Names Quilt, 53
narrative, 192
  see also talking about the dead;
    talking about the death
Nash, D., 85
national identity, 49
Newburn, T., 94
normal grief, 156, 157–8, 164–5

normalizing of emotions, 160, 162
Northern Ireland, 42, 46
  Protestant/Catholic differences, 146
nostalgia, 65, 66
numbness, 144–5

obituaries, 80–2
Oklahoma City bombing, 123
older bereaved people, 47, 52, 74
organ transplants, 86
organizational needs, 165
oscillation, 22, 27, 36, 52, 145, 147

palliative care, 50, 100
Palmer, L., 172–3
paranormal, 112
parent losing a child, 59, 71, 72, 107,
    108, 123
  gender of mourner, 172, 174, 176
  loss of a baby, 179
  loss of adult child, 81
  loss of soldier son, 44, 56, 88–94
  mutual help groups, 189–90
  reaction by others, 130, 191
  see also abortion; Compassionate
    Friends, The; miscarriage
Parkes, C., 64, 103–6, 171, 199–200
  explanation for sense of presence, 65
  gender differences, 175, 178
  normality, 157
  phases of grief, 161
  review of *Continuing Bonds*, 106,
    110
participant observation, *see*
    ethnography
pathological grief, *see* abnormal grief
pathologists, 98–9
patriarchy, 123
Pennells, M., 158
phases of grief, *see* stages of grief
photographs, 62–3, 94
Pike, C., 58
pilgrimage to war graves, 77, 94
Pincus, L., 105
police, 96
policing grief, 119–26, 202–3
  in family, 1–6
  gender, 123

pollution, 28
  and gender, 28
pop songs, 52
Porter, M., 154
Porter, R., 85
postmodernism, 111–12, 166, 186–7,
  206–8
post-mortems, *see* autopsies
post-traumatic stress disorder (PTSD),
  39, 45
power, 26, 30, 32
Prince, L., 72
Prior, L., 146
privacy
  of the dead, 81–2
  of mourners, *see* privatization of grief
privatization of grief, 31, 35–6, 54,
  143–6
  conflict with legal procedures, 96
progress, 112
property
  basis of funeral ritual, 30
  destruction of after death, 26
Protestantism, 32–4, 110, 112–13,
  128, 135
  see also Reformation, the
psycho-social transition theory, 104,
  110
Puckle, B., 131
Puff Daddy, 52
purgatory, 12–13, 32
puritans, 128

rationality, 110–13
Rees, D., 57, 65
reflexivity, 70, 125, 127
regulation, xiii, 120–1, 131, 193–4,
  203, 205–6
  over-regulation, 122–3
  self-regulation, 124–5
  under-regulation, 124, 142–3
  see also anomie; policing grief
Reformation, the, 32–3, 177
  deathbed accounts, 85
relics, 32
religious beliefs
  and deathbed accounts, 85
  in modern western societies, 12–13

and psychological explanations,
  27–8
  in traditional societies, 25–6
  see also ancestors; Catholicism;
  Judaism; Protestantism
remembrance, 42–4
reminder theory, 27–8, 65, 147
reminiscence work, 41
research methods, *see* ethnography;
  feminist methodology;
  methodological agnosticism
resolution of grief, 156, 198–9
reunion in heaven, 35, 47, 57–8
Richardson, R., 142
Riches, G., 63, 96, 176, 193–5
risk, 133–4
rites of passage, 28–9
ritual, 139–40
  see also funerals; rites of passage
road traffic accidents, 71, 95–6
Rock, P., 160
Rodgers, B., 164
romantic love, 34–7, 51, 111
Romantic Movement, 34–7, 51, 111,
  128, 132
romanticising the past, 23
Rose, N., 195–6
Rosenblatt, P., 27–8, 65, 119
Rossetti, C., 39, 127
Rubin, S., 199

Scheper-Hughes, N., 120
Schut, H., 182
  see also dual process model
Seale, C., 70, 98, 107, 165
searching, 65
Second World War, *see* World War
  Two
self, *see* identity; individualism
self help groups, *see* mutual help
  groups
sensing the presence of the dead, 8, 57,
  65
sentimentality, culture of, 112
separation of home and work, 71
shaman, 24
Shapiro, E., 52–3, 152
shiva, 29

sibling loss, 58, 72, 87
Silverman, D., 98
Silverman, P.
  continuing bonds, 105, 110
  research with widows, 27, 29, 123,
    145, 148, 172, 175–6, 193
Simonds, W., 123, 134, 156, 160, 162,
    172, 174, 178–80
Small, K., 93
Smith, Adam, 21, 128–30, 149, 180, 190
Soane, Sir John, 128–9
social class, 35, 130–1
social death, 49–50
social fragmentation, 73
social isolation, 75–6, 174, 194
social order, 98
social solidarity, xiii, 21–2, 128–30
Sora (India), 24
South Africa, 44
Soviet Union, 44
spiritual pain, 86, 101–2
spiritualism, 35, 44, 59–60, 132
spirituality, 57–60
stages of grief, 161–4
stiff upper lip, see emotional reserve;
    stoicism
stillbirths, 146
stoicism, 40–2, 132–4
storytelling, 70–1, 78–82
  ethics of, 80–2
Stroebe, M., 200
  dual process model, 22, 65, 145,
    163–4
  gender differences, 173–4
  grief theories, 110–12, 169–70
  grief work, evidence for, 160–1
student bereavement, 77
subculture, 191–2, 194
sudden death, 94–100
Sudnow, D., 98
suffering, 200
suicide, 87
  attempts, 12–13
  bereavement by, 58, 84, 107
  thoughts of, 66
suing, 100
suttee, 170
sympathy, see Smith, Adam

Tallensi (Ghana), 25–6
Tallis, Thomas, 127
talking about the dead, 8, 69–83
  barriers to, 72–5
  implications for professionals,
    78–82
  in mutual help groups, 191
  rules against, 70
talking about the death, 84–102
  implications for professionals,
    98–100
  official cover-ups, 93, 94–5, 100
  see also deathbed accounts
talking to the dead, 8, 11, 15, 60–1
  and gender, 61
tasks of grief, 158–9, 161
tears, see crying
theories of grief, 103–15
  modern, 110–11
  postmodern, 111–12
  revolution in, 108–13
therapy, 195–6
  see also counselling
Titanic, the, 81
Torrie, M., 158, 196
total pain, 100, 101–2
traditional societies, 23–32, 185–6
tragedy, see disasters
Troubridge, Lady, 143
Truth and Reconciliation Commission,
    46, 80, 100
Turner, V., 28

unfinished business, 86
Unruh, D., 56, 63
USA
  California, 150
  low cremation rate, 48–9
  military, 93
  religiosity, 58

van Gennep, A., 28–9, 107–8
veterans associations, 43
Victorian mourning, 34–7, 178
  rejection of, 36–7, 122, 130–1
Vietnam Veterans Memorial, 45, 62,
    172–3
Vietnam War, 45, 94

Vincent-Buffault, A., 134
Vitebsky, P., 24

Walter, T., New Model of Grief, 115
Wambach, J., 125, 162–3, 193
war, 39–46, 132–4
  civil, 42, 46
  graves, 42, 77
  letters from soldiers, 40, 44, 88–94
  memorials, 43, 44, 45, 62, 94
  remembrance, 42–4
Weiss, R., 71
widowers, 76
  compared to widows, 173–6
  depression, 173–4
  isolation, 76, 173–4
  remarriage, 76, 141, 174, 176–7
  work as distraction, 146–7
widows, 64, 75–7, 123
  compared to widowers, 173–6
  coping, 178
  Hindu, 170
  idealization of husband, *see*
    idealization
  over-researched, 171
  relationship with children, 145,
    177
  remarriage, 52, 76–7
  talking about the death, 84

Victorian, 35–6
wife to widow to woman, 29, 108,
  193
work as distraction, 27, 52, 146–7,
  176, 178
Wikan, U., 140
Wilkinson, A., 55
Williams, R., 29, 52
Winston's Wish, 85–6
Winter, J., 39–40, 43, 44, 93–4
women, 171–84
  connectedness, 113, 175
  deathbed spirituality, 85
  leisure to grieve, 35–6
  official keeners, 119–20
  pollution, 28
  rejection of Victorian mourning,
    36–7, 122, 130–1
  voice, 113, 178–9
  see also parent losing a child;
    widows
Worden, W., 109, 158–9, 161
working through grief, *see* grief, work
World War One, 37, 43, 44, 47,
  88–94, 142
World War Two, 41, 44
Wortman, C., 154, 160, 169–70

Young, M., 58

REFLECTIONS ON PALLIATIVE CARE

David Clark and Jane Seymour

Palliative care seems set to continue its rapid development into the early years of the twenty-first century. From its origins in the modern hospice movement, the new multidisciplinary specialty of palliative care has expanded into a variety of settings. Palliative care services are now being provided in the home, in hospital and in nursing homes. There are moves to extend palliative care beyond its traditional constituency of people with cancer. Efforts are being made to provide a wide range of palliative therapies to patients at an early stage of their disease progression. The evidence-base of palliative care is growing, with more research, evaluation and audit, along with specialist pro-grammes of education. Palliative care appears to be coming of age.

On the other hand numbers of challenges still exist. Much service develop-ment has been unplanned and unregulated. Palliative care providers must continue to adapt to changing patterns of commissioning and funding ser-vices. The voluntary hospice movement may feel its values threatened by a new professionalism and policies which require its greater integration within main-stream services. There are concerns about the re-medicalization of palliative care, about how an evidence-based approach to practice can be developed, and about the extent to which its methods are transferring across diseases and settings.

Beyond these preoccupations lie wider societal issues about the organization of death and dying in late modern culture. To what extent have notions of death as a contemporary taboo been superseded? How can we characterize the nature of suffering? What factors are involved in the debate surrounding end of life care ethics and euthanasia?

David Clark and Jane Seymour, drawing on a wide range of sources, as well as their own empirical studies, offer a set of reflections on the development of palliative care and its place within a wider social context. Their book will be essential reading to any practitioner, policy maker, teacher or student involved in palliative care or concerned about death, dying and life-limiting illness.

Contents
Introduction – Part 1: Death in society – The social meaning of death and suffering – Ageing, dying and grieving – The ethics of dying – Part II: The philosophy and practice of palliative care – History and development – Defini-tions, components, meanings – Routinization and medicalization – Part III: Policy issues – Policy development and palliative care – The delivery of palliat-ive care services – Part IV: Conclusion – The future for palliative care – References – Index.

224pp   0 335 19454 0 (Paperback)   0 335 19455 9 (Hardback)